ESSENTIALS OF TELEMEDICINE AND TELECARE

To Jo:
from whom any distance is too far

ESSENTIALS OF TELEMEDICINE AND TELECARE

A. C. NORRIS
*Department of Management Science and Information Systems,
University of Auckland, New Zealand*

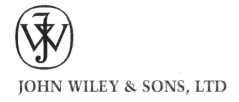

JOHN WILEY & SONS, LTD

Copyright © 2002 by John Wiley & Sons, Ltd
Baffins Lane, Chichester,
West Sussex PO19 1UD, England

National   01243 779777
International (+44) 1243 779777
e-mail (for orders and customer service enquiries): cs-books@wiley.co.uk
Visit our Home Page on http://www.wiley.co.uk
or http://www.wiley.com

Other Wiley Editorial Offices

John Wiley & Sons, Inc., 605 Third Avenue,
New York, NY 10158-0012, USA

WILEY-VCH Verlag GmbH, Pappelallee 3,
D-69469 Weinheim, Germany

John Wiley & Sons Australia Ltd, 33 Park Road, Milton,
Queensland 4064, Australia

John Wiley & Sons (Asia) Pte Ltd, 2 Clementi Loop #02-01,
Jin Xing Distripark, Singapore 129809

John Wiley & Sons (Canada) Ltd, 22 Worcester Road,
Rexdale, Ontario M9W 1L1, Canada

Library of Congress Cataloging-in-Publication Data

Norris, A. C. (Anthony Charles)
    Essentials of telemedicine and telecare / A.C. Norris.
      p. cm.
    Includes bibliographical references and index.
    ISBN 0-471-53151-0 (pbk)
      1. Telecommunication in medicine. I. Title.

    R119.9 .N67 2001
    362.1'028—dc21

                                                                    2001045411

British Library Cataloguing in Publication Data

A catalogue record for this book is available from the British Library

ISBN 0-471-53151-0

Typeset in 10/12pt Times by Mayhew Typesetting, Rhayader, Powys
Printed and bound in Great Britain by TJ International, Padstow, Cornwall
This book is printed on acid-free paper responsibly manufactured from sustainable forestry, in which at least two trees are planted for each one used for paper production.

CONTENTS

PREFACE

This book describes developments in the delivery of remote healthcare. If we regard telemedicine as simply the delivery of medicine at a distance, then the technique has been available since the invention of the telegraph and the telephone in the second half of the 19th century. However, the real technical drivers have been telecommunications and information technologies and their convergence as we enter the 21st century. Television and digital communications have been major forces in these developments.

Alongside the technical advances has come a concern to provide high-quality, expert healthcare where it is needed rather than to confine it to fixed points such as city hospitals or general practitioners' surgeries. Thus, we see better healthcare becoming available to rural and disadvantaged communities, to travellers, to people confined to their own homes, and to military personnel in theatres of war.

The text sets out to explain the main features of telemedicine and telecare and to reveal the potential of the new methodologies while keeping a watchful eye on their limitations and the barriers to progress. Many observers get distracted by the hyperbole surrounding robotic surgery across continents and the like—hopefully, we avoid falling into this trap.

Chapter 1 starts with a look at alternative definitions of telemedicine and why these have arisen. It constructs a definition that is concise but informative and then proposes similar definitions for telecare and telehealth. With these statements to guide our way, the chapter traces the origins and development of telemedicine, and then looks at the technological, clinical and business drivers that have led advances throughout the world.

Chapter 2 identifies the main types of telemedicine and considers how they influence patients and carers. The second part of this chapter records the benefits derived from remote healthcare but then focuses the watchful eye on the inherent limitations and the external barriers to progress. These benefits, limitations and barriers are never far from the surface throughout the rest of the book.

In Chapter 3, we examine the technology of telemedicine, starting with an understanding of the types of data we may need to transfer across the telemedicine link. These types determine the nature of the videoconferencing equipment we use and the hardware and software needed to maintain the accuracy and utility of transmitted images. After a consideration of some essential communication protocols, we round off the chapter with an overview of the main telecommunication standards that ensure the interoperability of equipment and the valid transmission and receipt of data.

Chapter 4 switches attention to the people who use the technology and how they use it. It looks at public and private healthcare providers and distinguishes fixed-point applications, such as those typically based on specialities found in acute hospitals, and mobile applications such as ambulance services and disaster recovery.

Chapter 5 describes how to set up and operate a telemedicine service. The emphasis is on the critical success factors. Thus, the chapter first directs attention to the strategic context that arises from government policy and how it constrains the project. It then takes the reader through the process of evaluating pilot studies before looking at defining needs, making the business case, and developing and operating a mainstream service.

The final chapter, Chapter 6, addresses the ethical and legal issues associated with telemedicine. These issues include duty and standards of care, confidentiality and security, rights of access, malpractice, physician licensure and reimbursement, and intellectual property rights. A section is devoted to the ethical and legal aspects of healthcare advice and provision on the Internet. We can do no more than touch the surface of a very involved subject here but we try to give the reader the knowledge to avoid the most obvious pitfalls and to understand new developments as they come along.

The book aims to give an understanding of the main features of telemedicine and the issues surrounding its development and use. It tries to provide a good working knowledge of the subject matter together with an in-depth survey of literature where the reader can find the detail omitted from the text.

References are mainly cited to primary sources, journal papers and textbooks. Sometimes, however, it is more convenient for readers to access a summary or other version from the Internet and so URLs to such sources are added wherever possible to supplement original publications. Readers will appreciate that URLs are less permanent than traditional published sources and that the author and publishers have no control over the addition, modification or removal of these links, which may not always return the required information. All cited links were active at the end of January 2001. There is also an annotated book list and guide to web sites.

Tony Norris
Department of Management Science and Information Systems
University of Auckland

1

ORIGINS AND DEVELOPMENT

OBJECTIVES

At the end of this chapter you should be able to:

- understand why there are different definitions of telemedicine;
- trace the origins and development of telemedicine;
- identify the technological and non-technological drivers of telemedicine;
- recognise the influence of funding on telemedicine development;
- appreciate how telemedicine is used in developed and underdeveloped nations;
- suggest key directions for the future of telemedicine.

1.1 INTRODUCTION

Chapter 1 provides an overview of telemedicine, its origins, acceptance and adoption throughout the world.

It is always useful to clarify the boundaries of our discussion and so we start with a look at the terms *telemedicine* and *telecare*. Over the years these terms have changed (and continue to change) their meaning and it is instructive to see why this is so. The analysis also helps us to establish working definitions for the remainder of the book.

The chapter then goes on to review the origins of telemedicine and the reasons for the upsurge of interest since the early 1990s. This review allows us to identify the technological and non-technological drivers of development. The effect of funding on telemedicine projects is also examined to see how it influences project choice and sustainability.

The different drivers of development also give us an insight into the distribution of projects throughout the world, and the chapter continues with a brief survey of telemedicine in developed and underdeveloped countries.

Finally, we try to spot the trends that will shape the future of telemedicine and telecare.

1.2   DEFINITIONS OF TELEMEDICINE, TELEHEALTH AND TELECARE

1.2.1   Telemedicine

The prefix *tele* derives from the Greek meaning 'far' or 'at a distance' or 'remote'. Hence the word *telemedicine* signifies:

> medicine delivered at a distance.

This definition suggests that telemedicine is restricted to the treatment of patients by clinicians, a constraint that has become less true with the development of telemedical practice. Beyond this suggestion the definition is quite uninformative since it gives no clue as to how to deliver medicine at a distance. A more accurate and informative definition of telemedicine is therefore [1]:

> the transfer of electronic medical data from one location to another.

This definition at least implies the use of information and telecommunication technologies to make the transfer, and replacement of the word 'medicine' by the term 'transfer of medical data' removes the restriction to patient treatment. At the same time, the breadth of this new definition says nothing about the purpose of the transfer. So can we do better? Here is a 1995 definition that gives more detail in just a few more words [2]:

> Telemedicine is the use of telecommunications to provide medical information and services.

We are now made aware of the role of telecommunications (but not necessarily information technology) and we know that the provision of medical information (assumed to be synonymous with data) and services are the goals of the telecommunications link.

But why are we providing these services? A 1999 definition adopted for a Congressional briefing on telemedicine in the USA produces a statement that is even more informative without being verbose [3]:

> Telemedicine utilizes information and telecommunications technology to transfer medical information for diagnosis, therapy and education.

Treatment is clearly stated as a prime objective but so is education, revealing an increasingly common role for telemedicine, one that is not directly associated with treatment.

If we want even more information then we can separately explain the terms of the definition without damaging its conciseness. For example, we can observe that the technology may simply be a telephone or a facsimile machine although the use of information technology suggests that more often than not there is some computer involvement.

The medical information may include images, live video and audio, video and sound files, patient medical records, and output data from medical devices. The transfer may involve interactive video and audio communication between patients and medical professionals, or between those professionals without patient participation. Alternatively, it may simply describe the transmission of patient data either from monitoring devices (*telemetry*) or from medical histories (electronic patient records). Those taking part in the transfer may be located in a GP surgery, a hospital clinic or some other environment if the occasion is an emergency (e.g. after an accident).

1.2.2 Telehealth

We have arrived at an acceptable definition of telemedicine but there are many others based on lengthier statements and even longer explanations. A fascinating analysis of several alternatives is contained in a scoping study of telemedicine for the Australian Commonwealth Department of Industry, Science and Tourism [4]. The study concludes that the term 'telemedicine' is gradually going out of favour and being replaced by *telehealth*.

The rationale for this shift in emphasis arises from changing practice. Thus, until the mid-1990s, most telemedicine links involved medical doctor consultations using telecommunications to bridge the distance. The transfer of medical information was the immediate goal of such links.

More recently, however, other health professionals such as community workers and psychologists have become involved and the term 'telehealth' has been coined to describe this expansion beyond the confines of clinical medicine. Although experience and changes in practice are at the root of this shift, it has been accelerated by falling costs and increased access to equipment, as well as by more general facilities such as the Internet [4].

Developing our concepts, we can now define telehealth according to the statement:

> Telehealth is the use of information and communication technologies to transfer healthcare information for the delivery of clinical, administrative and educational services.

Extension to include administrative healthcare information recognises the use of telematic services to transfer demographic and operational information that may have little or no clinical content. Similarly, while distance learning courses for healthcare professionals are covered by the banner of telehealth, components of these courses may concentrate on health policy or other non-clinical topics.

1.2.3   Telecare

By convention, the term 'telemedicine' is usually confined to remote medicine in primary and secondary care, and emergency locations. In contrast, the term *telecare* is often used to describe the application of telemedicine to deliver medical services to patients in their own homes or supervised institutions. Telecare is regarded as distinct from telemedicine because it is especially important for a specific group of patients with long-term chronic conditions such as mental illness, disability or simply old age, which reduce their freedom of movement.

Naturally, our definitions of telemedicine and telehealth could encompass telecare since neither says anything about location. The more common approach, however, is to define telecare separately, as follows:

> Telecare utilises information and communication technologies to transfer medical information for the diagnosis and therapy of patients in their place of domicile.

1.2.4   Summary of Working Definitions and E-Health

We now have several statements that we can harmonise as working definitions for use throughout this book. Here we go!

- *Telemedicine*: use of information and communication technologies to transfer medical information for the delivery of clinical and educational services.
- *Telehealth*: the use of information and communication technologies to transfer healthcare information for the delivery of clinical, administrative and educational services.
- *Telecare*: the use of information and communication technologies to transfer medical information for the delivery of clinical services to patients in their place of domicile.

Notice how the definitions say nothing about the nature of the medicine involved. As we shall see, certain medical disciplines are more suitable for telemedical activity than others, but telemedicine is not new medicine. It is rather a new way of delivering existing medicine, extending distance and access.

Our definitions are not necessarily the 'best of breed' but they are accurate, coherent, informative and up to date—not a bad set of attributes.

A moment's thought will reveal a further connection between the definitions, namely that telemedicine and telecare can be regarded as subsets of telehealth. In this book we are concerned mainly with the level at which telemedicine and, to a lesser extent, telecare are practised and these are the definitions we shall use most. A further debate is concerned with whether telemedicine is a subset of medical informatics [5].

An alternative hierarchy has been proposed in another report for the Australian Government, which argues that telehealth applications that make use of Internet technologies should be regarded as examples of *e-health*, a subset of e-commerce [6]. This terminology is gaining ground at present [7] as a component of the 'e-everything' bandwagon. The current use of the term is, however, confusing. Some protagonists use it to include all aspects of telemedicine; others confine it to the use of the Internet (by e-patients and e-physicians!) to access healthcare information [8]. Elsewhere the term seems to have more to do with slick marketing than useful categorisation. We shall use it sparingly.

1.3 ORIGINS AND DEVELOPMENT OF TELEMEDICINE

1.3.1 From Beginnings to Modern Times

A glance at any article or book on telemedicine will reveal so many different versions of the history of the technique and different dates for the same event[1] that you begin to wonder if anyone really knows how it all began and developed. The confusion arises because telemedicine was not invented as a well-defined discipline with specialised instrumentation and protocols. Clinicians simply appropriated and began to use new technologies developed for other purposes as they became available. Take-up was therefore piecemeal and uncoordinated.

Neglecting the use of bonfires to alert mediaeval populations to the spread of bubonic plague and the postal system to send medical data [9] (both excluded by our definition), we can identify four phases of telemedicine development based on the exploitation of telecommunication and information technologies. These are shown in Table 1.1.

Let us look at some examples from the different phases that chart the progress and advances in telemedicine to the present day.

Telegraphy was used during the American Civil War to send casualty lists and order supplies [10] but it was rapidly replaced as a means of long-distance communication following Marconi's invention of the radio-telegraph in 1897 [11]. Until the end of the first quarter of the 20th century, sea voyages were the principal means of long-distance, international travel and the 1920s and 1930s saw the introduction of several *radio-medical* services (the radio phase). In one form or another, these services continue in operation to the present day. The most celebrated example is the Italian International Radio Medicine

---

[1] There is sometimes ambiguity in dates as one author cites the start of a project and another states the date of publication of the results.

Table 1.1.   Main phases of telemedicine development

Development phase	Approximate timescale
Telegraphy and telephony	1840s–1920s
Radio	1920s onwards (main technology until 1950s)
Television/space technologies	1950s onwards (main technology until 1980s)
Digital technologies	1990s onwards

Centre, which began in 1935 and had assisted over 42,000 patients, mainly seafarers, by 1996 [11].

The next phase of development coincided with the widespread availability of black-and-white television in the 1950s. The ability to visualise a patient's condition rather than rely on an audio description greatly enhanced diagnosis and the confidence of those engaged in treatment.

From a closed-circuit television service begun in 1955, the Nebraska Psychiatric Institute developed a two-way link with Norfolk State Hospital, 112 miles away, in 1964 with further extensions in 1971 [12]. The links were used for education and consultations between consultants and GPs. This project is one of the first of many examples of telepsychiatry.

Also begun in the late 1950s was a 20-year collaboration between Lockheed, the US Public Health Service and the National Aeronautics and Space Administration (NASA). The project, Space Technology Applied to Rural Papago Advanced Health Care (STARPAHC), sought to provide medical care to rural communities of Papago Indians in Arizona via the transmission of electrocardiographs and X-rays to centres staffed by specialists [13].

This was one of the first examples of teleradiology, pioneered in Canada in 1957 by Dr Albert Jutras [14], and one of the first uses of telemedicine to extend the reach of conventional services to rural or disadvantaged communities.

The STARPAHC project demonstrates another important contribution to the development of telemedicine, namely the impetus to research and development given by various space programmes in the 1960s and in particular by America's NASA. In the late 1960s, NASA also pioneered significant advances in telemetry [13] as the Agency sought to understand the effects of zero gravity on blood pressure, respiration rate, ECG and so on.

A less adventurous type of traveller was catered for by the Logan International Airport facility set up in 1967 to provide occupational health services to airport employees and to deliver emergency care and medical attention to air passengers [15]. A microwave link connected the airport clinic with Massachusetts General Hospital, and, along with the Nebraska Institute project mentioned above, the project was one of the earliest instances of physician–patient interaction using two-way interactive television (IATV).

In the 1970s the first batch of commercial communications satellites became available, and clinicians quickly saw the opportunities to extend the scope of telemedicine. Again, North America was the scene of the main activity. Examples include the Alaska Satellite Biomedical Demonstration Program to improve village healthcare [16], and various Canadian projects to serve remote areas based upon NASA's Hermes satellite, launched in 1976 [11, 17].

Two programmes from the 1980s illustrate the increasing sophistication of visioning facilities, including the use of colour, and the extension of satellite links to emergency situations as opposed to those with established and permanent connections. The first is the North-West Telemedicine Project set up in Queensland, Australia, the only major telemedicine project outside North America until 1990. This project was designed to serve rural communities, including Aborigine populations [18]. It offered an alternative to the Flying Doctor service and prompted one of the first serious attempts to evaluate a telemedicine programme for cost effectiveness.

The second example is the NASA SpaceBridge to Armenia set up in the wake of the terrible earthquake in December 1988 [1]. SpaceBridge allowed video, voice and facsimile consultations to take place between specialist centres in the USA and a medical centre in Yerevan, Armenia, thereby providing the first truly international telemedicine programme.

These are just a few representative examples to show the development of telemedicine up until the modern era. Further information is available in the publications cited and in the report by Grigsby and Kaehny [19].

1.3.2   Modern Telemedicine and Telecare

The momentum in telemedicine research and development built comparatively slowly until the end of the 1980s, at which point it began to accelerate rapidly. The main reasons for this increase in pace are considered in Section 1.4 but the transition from analogue to digital communications and the accompanying role of computers and information technologies such as mobile telephones were clearly major drivers.

At the same time, the lead taken by the USA since the early days of telemedicine has been maintained so that over 50% of the primary research is now conducted in the USA compared with 40% in the whole of Europe and around 10% in Asia and Australasia [10].

Thus, since the mid-1990s we have seen telemedicine invade more and more clinical specialities and increase the total number of consultations. For example, in the USA, Allen and Grigsby report that nearly 40 000 teleconsultations were performed in 1998 in more than 35 different specialties [20]. Around 70% of the episodes used interactive video, the rest using prerecorded or non-video technologies.

The number of teleconsultations is, of course, small compared with the total number of consultations by conventional face-to-face methods. The figures exclude teleradiology, which remains the single most popular (and prerecorded) application with more than 250 000 consultations in the USA alone in 1997 [10]. This latter number reflects the long-term standing of teleradiology as one of the few telemedicine specialities that has entered mainstream healthcare. As a consequence, teleradiology receives full reimbursement under the USA's Medicare healthcare scheme.

Since 1994 we have also seen the phenomenal rise of interest in the Internet, not just as a source of information (tele-education), but as a means of communication. Streaming audio and video raise the prospect of remote consultation via the superhighway, provided bandwidth issues can be addressed and security problems overcome.

The survey of origins and progress in Section 1.3 suggests some of the parameters that are driving the development of telemedicine and telecare. Let us draw these out more clearly and set the scene for more detailed discussion at a later stage.

1.4   DRIVERS OF TELEMEDICINE AND TELECARE

1.4.1   Technological Drivers

We can identify three main drivers under this heading:

- computing and information technology;
- network and telecommunications infrastructure;
- technology-led society.

The following subsections comment briefly on the features that apply to telemedicine. Chapter 3 looks at the technology of telemedicine in more detail.

Computing and Information Technology

We have already mentioned the transition from analogue to digital communications and the accompanying role of computing. As in almost every other walk of life, each development in IT expands access, improves existing services and leads to new facilities. Falling equipment costs, increased power on the desktop and ease-of-use are important factors in the progress of telemedicine, as are modern developments in videoconferencing.

Of equal importance, however, is the increase in the reliability of equipment [21]. As Chapter 3 shows, telemedicine systems consist of multiple components, often operating unattended over large distances, and involving many switching, analogue–digital, and vision–sound–electrical signal conversions. With so many interfaces, there are frequent opportunities for equipment incompatibility and malfunction, and no telemedicine system will remain in use for long unless it is as reliable as conventional alternatives.

Network and Telecommunications Infrastructure

Naturally, it is not just the power on the desktop that drives the advance of IT but the ability to share information over local and wide area computer networks. The development and convergence of communications technologies, and the bewildering array of new transmission protocols, have led to major improvements and opportunities in telemedicine services, as in many other areas of information exchange.

Low-performance, modem technologies based on copper wire transmission have been supplemented by faster media and technologies using fibre-optic cables. The installation of national fibre-optic (T1, T3) backbones (e.g. the NSFNET and its successors in the USA [22]) has promoted an expansion of telemedicine services in several countries.

Even so, the need for greater bandwidth has led to the introduction of new protocols such as asymmetric digital subscriber line (ADSL) and asynchronous transfer mode (ATM), and major developments in wireless and satellite technologies [23]. Several of these broadband technologies are competing for attention, a fact that will inevitably lead to lower prices and added value.

Technology-Led Society

The pace of technological change feeds on the appetite of society for ever greater speed, convenience and quality [24, 25]. Nowhere is this appetite so voracious as in the USA, which has been the kitchen for innovation and progress in technology in general, and information technology in particular. Microsoft, IBM, Intel, Motorola, CISCO, Netscape and Sun Microsystems are just a few of the chefs that come to mind.

The USA's national taste for technology is coupled with other national characteristics, e.g. an aptitude to develop strategy on an expansive scale ('think big') and organise resources to implement the strategies (the 'can do' or 'no problem' philosophies). National space and defence programmes are typical examples. The development and role of medical technology is another, more pertinent, illustration.

As a consequence, the USA has been at the forefront of advances in telemedicine, not just in research but in the all-important follow-up of moving telemedicine into the healthcare mainstream (see Section 5.2).

1.4.2   Non-Technological Drivers

Non-technological drivers can be just as important as those that harness technology. We can distinguish seven key factors that have helped, and are helping, the development of telemedicine:

- extension of access to healthcare service;
- healthcare provision for travellers;
- military applications;
- home telecare;
- cost reduction;
- market development;
- health policy and strategy.

Extension of Access to Healthcare Services

Extending healthcare access to individuals and communities who have limited, erratic or negligible access to such services has motivated telemedicine developers from the earliest times to the present day. Beneficiaries include patients who live in rural areas with few healthcare professionals to look after them, and residents who inhabit areas that are cut off from normal transport at certain times of the year by bad weather. Isolated communities in parts of Australia and the USA provide examples of the former, as does Canada, which also provides an exemplar of climatic difficulties.

Telemedicine services can overcome the 'tyranny of distance' presented by these conditions and reduce medical and economic risks [2].

However, deprivation of healthcare services is not confined to those who choose to live outside of urban areas and the concentration of medical facilities. Telemedical services are now on offer to the occupants of penal [26] and mental institutions, thereby avoiding the costs and dangers of transporting patients to external health facilities.[2]

As we have seen, a similar rationale lies behind the provision of telecare services to elderly or handicapped people in their own homes.

Healthcare Provision for Travellers

Even members of the public who live within permanent access of first-level medical services may find themselves denied such assistance on their travels. We are all travelling further and more often, so healthcare while 'in transit' is assuming greater importance.

The classical predicament arises at sea [27] where modern crewing levels make it likely that no crew member possesses more than rudimentary first-aid experience. Radio-medicine (Section 1.3.1) has long been the first back-up system in these circumstances, providing advice either for treatment or for diverting the voyage and heading for a port with the required facilities.

Telemedicine can do better although it cannot, of course, increase the expertise of crew members. However, transmission of ECG or blood pressure

---

[2] User satisfaction surveys from prisoners are not encouraging!

readings from telemetric tests, or visual or X-ray images from a videoconferencing system, to a shore-based physician can improve diagnosis and lead to more appropriate care. It may also prevent an unnecessary (and possibly expensive or dangerous) diversion to port.

Similar problems can occur on flights—an increasingly common mode of travel (including astronauts). Over the year April 1993 to March 1994, British Airways (BA) dealt with 2078 medical incidents [27]. Fortunately, most of these were minor and related to air sickness but there was a significant number of serious incidents such as heart attacks and respiratory problems. BA staff are highly trained to deal with such emergencies but no commercial aircraft carries the personnel or medical equipment to set up an operating theatre.

The cost of diverting a Boeing 747 aeroplane is typically £40 000 so BA is actively looking at ways of using telemedicine to transmit vital signs and help cabin crew or passengers with medical experience to carry out possibly life-saving interventions.

Military Applications

Military applications are in a sense comparable to providing healthcare for travellers; patients are prevented from normal access to first-class medical facilities. However, the circumstances are quite different and the ratio of conventional disease to emergency conditions is often the reverse of that met in civilian life.

Furthermore, many of the emergencies are likely to be serious injuries incurred in conflict and of a different type (e.g. gunshot or explosion injuries) to those met in the civilian world. The priority to restore to health is coupled with the need to return the combatant to active duty as soon as possible. Telemedicine and videoconferencing are therefore seen to offer new and better opportunities for triage [28] and life-saving treatment involving film-less radiology and telesurgery where field surgeons are mentored in real time by consultant specialists [29].

Notwithstanding the emphasis on wounds and surgery, hostilities often occur in countries with different disease patterns from those normally experienced by NATO and UN troops. Soldiers are therefore exposed to diseases for which they have little immunity. Add to this the fear of chemical warfare, and Mobile Army Surgical Hospitals (MASH) and their equivalents have to be at the forefront of medical *tele*-technology.

The US army now operates the Primetime III network, described as a 'military medical Internet' [28], making it possible for troops in Bosnia to receive the same quality of care that they would get in the USA. The academic and industrial links formed during the development of Primetime III, and the test-bed experience gained, will undoubtedly fuel the next round of developments in conventional as well as military and emergency telemedicine.

Home Telecare

Telecare has also captured an increasing amount of attention since the mid-1990s as all developed nations face up to the problems posed by an ageing population. In 1998 there were 380 million people in the world aged over 65, a ratio of 10:1 for every new baby born [30]. By 2020 there will be more than 800 million people aged over 65, giving an elderly/new-born ratio of 15:1. Two-thirds of these over-65s will be in developing countries. In China alone the number of people over the age of 60 (274 million) will be higher than the total population of the United States.

The increase in the proportion of older people in the population also changes the profile of illness and increases the incidence of chronic, long-term conditions. The relevance of telecare is twofold; the majority of elderly people prefer to live their lives in their own homes, and health providers can reduce costs by providing home care instead of expensive hospitalisation [31].

At the same time, it may be possible to replace some of the home visits by tele-visits in which a home-health nurse converses with a patient by a video link and receives up-to-date information and vital signs, especially if these patients live in rural or remote areas. This approach forms the monitoring basis of a very successful renal dialysis project at the Queen Elizabeth Hospital in Adelaide, South Australia [32, 33].

In other circumstances, the nurse could spend more time with needy patients or see more patients in a day. Alternatively, the hospital management may see opportunities for reducing the number of nursing staff to save salaries and overheads.

Cost Reduction

As suggested above, many healthcare providers have become interested in telemedicine as a means of cutting running costs. Health maintenance organisations (HMOs) in the USA are driving hard to realise these savings.

HMOs and physician–hospital alliances in many parts of the USA are competing for regional contracts to provide healthcare services on the basis of cost, quality and access to care [34]. The combination of increased competition, mandated access to care and increased provider risk related to patient outcomes is making these providers look carefully at telemedicine technologies. In particular, telemedicine is perceived as a tool to reduce the medical and economic risks associated with delivering healthcare to patients in rural areas (see above) and to provide remote, low-cost speciality services where full-time staffing is impractical [2].

Very few telemedicine projects have carried out rigorous cost–benefit evaluations or demonstrated the cost effectiveness of telemedicine services. A survey by Allen and Stein of several studies across a range of medical disciplines and applications concludes that general teleradiology, telepsychiatry, and home and prison telecare are most likely to be cost effective [35].

We shall return to this issue several times throughout the book.

Market Development

Despite the comparatively low capital costs of telemedical equipment, the uncertain operational costs have made it difficult to demonstrate overall cost benefits. As a consequence, the market for telemedicine suppliers has yet to take off. These same suppliers have therefore taken to driving the market to get it up to speed.

Telecommunications providers have had a particularly hard time. In an analogue world they could offer speciality services such as telephone calls, television programming etc. Now they are selling essentially the same commodity—digital bandwidth [2]. To survive they must therefore either increase the size of the overall market or differentiate their product from the competition. They judge that telemedicine can do both; hence their interest in promoting the technology, particularly in user-friendly areas such as telecare.

Health Policy and Strategy

Policy makers were late to get on board the telemedicine bandwagon. There were occasional, comforting statements from official sources but rarely were these more than attempts to demonstrate that the authorities were up to date and the public could safely leave healthcare in their competent hands. Until quite recently, therefore, policy statements have done little to shape or coordinate telemedicine development.

This situation seems set to change. We have already mentioned (Section 1.2.1) the Congressional briefing on telehealth in the USA, which will undoubtedly lead to further government statements, and the policy advocating submissions to the Australian Commonwealth Department of Industry, Science and Tourism (Sections 1.2.2 and 1.2.4), which will have the same effect.

In the United Kingdom (UK), the new Labour government heralded the telemedical future in its 1997 White Paper *The New NHS* [36], and developed this theme in the 1998 information technology strategy, *Information for Health* [37]. These documents require health authorities to include telemedicine in their thinking and planning for future services so that policy sets the framework for local solutions—not quite the same thing as a centrally directed policy.

However, the most forward-looking telemedicine policy by far is to be found in Malaysia. In its endeavour to become a developed nation by 2020, the Malaysian government has embarked upon a Multimedia Super Corridor Programme [38], which has seven flagship projects destined to revolutionise government, business, education and health.

The health project begun in 1997 is entitled the *Telemedicine Flagship Application* [39] and, as with other projects within the programme, a legal framework of 'cyberlaws' has been drafted to encourage investment and facilitate the rapid development of infrastructure and IT solutions. Although slowed by the 1997 Asian financial crisis, the vision, strategy and implementation will undoubtedly achieve the project goals. The world looks on, and hopefully learns.

We return to policy and strategy issues in Sections 2.5 and 5.2.

1.4.3 The Funding Dilemma

Research funding has obviously been critical to the development of telemedicine and telecare. In North America many projects, both large and small, have been centred in academic institutions and funded by government via such bodies as the US National Library of Medicine. Telecommunications companies have also been involved. However, Perednia and Allen bemoan the fact that, with the exception of the 20-year old programme at the Memorial University of Newfoundland, none of the projects begun before 1986 has survived [2].

They attribute the demise of these projects to the difficulty of demonstrating cost benefits, although the discontinuous nature of technological developments and the low emphasis on change management and cultural factors may contribute to some of the failures.

A similar pattern is observed in the UK. The Telemedicine Information Service [40] located at the University of Portsmouth, and sponsored by the Department of Health and the British Library, lists a range of projects again centred on academic institutions or hospitals closely associated with academia. Most of these projects have been relatively small programmes funded by academic grants or with the support of the National Health Service. British Telecom has been a significant participant but has now reduced its involvement. Again, several projects have folded and there is little mainstream activity or dissemination of good practice.

European Union funding is also available to UK groups and their European partners via the Advanced Informatics in Medicine (AIM—DG XIII-C3) [41] component of the Telematics Programme. Several high-profile and substantial projects have been undertaken. These projects seem to concentrate on technical and data standards.

These remarks suggest that rather than being driven by research funding, telemedicine is being hindered by the lack of it and in particular by the absence of funding that is independent of the information communications industry [10]. In contrast, Malaysia and, to a lesser extent, Australia have taken the view that industry should be the main sponsoring partner in telemedicine development (as opposed to basic research).

There is therefore a dilemma and a debate as to whether telemedicine will advance from carrying out basic research supported from central funding or from development work sponsored by industry [42].

Now that we have traced the development of telemedicine and seen what drives it forward we can use the information we have gained to understand where and how telemedicine is practised.

1.5   TELEMEDICINE IN DEVELOPED AND UNDERDEVELOPED COUNTRIES

1.5.1   Developed Countries

Every developed nation throughout the world, whatever the political persuasion of its government, is facing serious difficulties with the delivery of healthcare to its citizens. This is the case whether government is federal or national, whether the main source of funding is taxation or insurance (social or private), or whether provision is mainly in the hands of the public or private sector.

The USA and the countries of Europe exhibit the full diversity of these different systems but they face the same daunting problems, particularly:

- the increasing age of the population;
- the increasing cost of medical technology;
- patient expectations;
- economic and social change.

These and other factors drive up the cost of healthcare and reduce equity of access. Governments have three main ways to address these problems: increase taxation (particularly in welfare systems), ration the provision of healthcare or make healthcare more cost effective. The first two options are politically sensitive and in several countries have currently been pressed to their practical limits. Increasingly, therefore, administrations are turning to the third alternative and seeking to control the cost of healthcare while improving its effectiveness and 'adding value' to meet patient expectations.

As we have seen, this goal of cost reduction is a major driver of interest in telemedicine, which offers the prospect of lower costs for providers, especially staffing and overheads, as well as reduced travel costs for patients. As we have also noted, the cost effectiveness of many projects has yet to be established beyond doubt.

At the same time, telemedicine is perceived to be more convenient for the patient, to extend access to communities, and to improve the quality of treatment by expanding specialist advice. These advantages are difficult to factor into the cost–benefit equation but they are attractive to countries such as Australia, Canada, Sweden, Norway and Finland where distance and/or climate prevent rural communities from experiencing the same provision of services as their urban counterparts.

1.5.2   Underdeveloped Countries

The priorities in underdeveloped countries are very different. Often finance, organisation, culture and/or distance do not allow the authorities to provide even basic healthcare. In such nations communicable diseases and deaths from childbirth claimed almost 80% of the 51 million deaths worldwide in 1993 [11]. Most of these deaths could be avoided by simple and inexpensive treatment if help in the form of vaccination, improved sanitation and access to clean water could be provided to the people who need it.

Life expectancy in the developed world is 78 years; in most of the under-developed nations it is 43 years. Telemedicine offers the hope of remote clinics identifying disease at the earliest possible stage, leading to the necessary treatment locally or at some specialised location when needed.

While underdeveloped countries are unable to finance these programmes themselves, a surprising amount of progress can be made with small clinics, voluntary organisations and satellite links to specialists in industrialised countries. Examples include Russia, and countries in South and Central America, Asia and Africa with links to the USA, Norway and other European nations [10].

1.6   THE FUTURE FOR TELEMEDICINE

You should now have a good idea of what telemedicine is, how it has developed, what drives advances and where it is practised. So what does this tell us about future trends? Here are a few points based on our discussion and from the US Congressional Hearing article [3] referred to earlier. See also [43].

- *Moving telemedicine into the mainstream.* Telemedicine will only move out of the pilot study phase and into the sustainable mainstream if it is seen to be cost effective. This means that it must demonstrably save money compared with equivalent, direct services or we must find new ways of quantifying elements such as expansion of access, quality of care, patient convenience etc.
- *Health policy and strategy.* The benefits of telemedicine will be delayed and reduced unless governments see telemedicine as a strategic tool and consider how it should figure in their primary, secondary and tertiary healthcare delivery. Telemedicine also has the potential to achieve better integration of care than is often the case at present.
- *Telecare.* Home telemedicine would appear to have a significant role to play given the ageing populations throughout the world. More work needs to be done on making equipment easy to use and unobtrusive, and the cultural aspects hold as many, if not more, problems as the technical ones.

- *The role of the Internet.* The Internet offers almost endless possibilities for the delivery of information and education to both carers and patients and for the empowerment of the latter group. The technology will go some way to redressing the all too unequal balance between physician and patient, and, if used properly, can help patients to be more closely involved in managing their own care. The Internet can also be used to transmit health information and images.
- *Enhancing healthcare in underdeveloped countries.* Developed countries, commercial companies and non-profit organisations can make a real contribution by assisting underdeveloped countries to establish and improve basic healthcare.

1.7 SUMMARY

In Chapter 1 we have seen that:

- There are many definitions of telemedicine, which reflect changes in the understanding and practice of telemedical techniques.
- Telemedicine is the use of information and communication technologies to transfer medical information for the delivery of clinical and educational services.
- Telehealth is the use of information and communication technologies to transfer healthcare information for the delivery of clinical, administrative and educational services.
- Telecare is the use of information and communication technologies to transfer medical information for the delivery of clinical services to patients in their place of domicile.
- We can divide the development of telemedicine into four phases: telegraphy and telephony, radio, television/space technologies, and digital technologies.
- Technological drivers of telemedicine development include computing and information technology, network and telecommunications infrastructure, and a technology-led society.
- Non-technological drivers include extension of access to healthcare services, healthcare provision for travellers, military applications, home telecare, cost reduction, market development, and health policy.
- There is a dilemma and a debate as to whether telemedicine will advance from carrying out basic research or from development work sponsored by industry.
- Developed nations adopt telemedicine and telecare to lower costs, increase convenience for patients, extend access to communities, and improve the quality of treatment by expanding specialist advice.

- In underdeveloped nations, telemedicine offers the hope of identifying disease at an early stage, leading to the necessary treatment locally or at some specialised location.
- Priorities for the future of telemedicine include moving telemedicine into the mainstream, development of health policy and strategy, telecare, exploiting the Internet, and enhancing healthcare in underdeveloped countries.

2

SCOPE, BENEFITS AND LIMITATIONS OF TELEMEDICINE

OBJECTIVES

At the end of this chapter you should be able to:

- distinguish between teleconsultation, telemonitoring, tele-education and telesurgery;
- understand the effect of telemedicine on patients and carers;
- identify the benefits and limitations of telemedicine;
- discuss important barriers to the development and adoption of tele-medicine.

2.1 INTRODUCTION

Chapter 2 deals with issues that practice has shown to be important when considering telemedicine as an appropriate means of healthcare delivery. How we should develop and deliver a service once the decision to use telemedicine has been made is considered in Chapter 5.

This chapter begins by distinguishing the various types of telemedicine that currently define its scope. Focusing on healthcare delivery, the chapter then looks at the central issue of how patients and carers are affected by tele-medical practice.

The discussion leads to a review of the benefits and limitations of tele-medicine. The disadvantages we acknowledge here are essentially operational ones that commonly arise in practice. Finally, we probe some more strategic barriers to telemedicine development that are inherent in current thinking about healthcare delivery.

Strategic, legal and ethical issues comprise a repeated theme throughout the book and we return to them in more detail in later chapters.

2.2 TYPES OF TELEMEDICINE

The scope and categorisation of telemedicine (and telecare) practice have changed as the technology has developed. Currently, we can identify four different types:

- teleconsultation;
- tele-education;
- telemonitoring;
- telesurgery.

The following subsections look at each of these categories and identify some of their features.

2.2.1 Teleconsultation

The medical consultation is at the heart of clinical practice. Not surprisingly, therefore, *teleconsultation* to support clinical decision making is the most frequent example of telemedical procedures. Studies have shown that teleconsultation accounts for about 35% of the usage of telemedicine networks [44]; the remaining time is devoted to tele-education and to administration.

A teleconsultation can take place between two or more carers without patient involvement or between one or more carers and a patient. The simplest example is a telephone conversation between two physicians to obtain a second opinion. The physicians may be in different rooms in the same building or in different countries over a satellite link.

The most frequent image of a teleconsultation, however, is of a patient and his or her doctor communicating via a videoconferencing link. This type of link usually takes place in *real time* to generate the interactive feedback (i.e. consultation) that acts upon information as it is received. The alternative *store-and-forward* technology is frequently used in teleradiology for the transmission of large X-ray files at periods of low network traffic. In these situations, the delay between receipt of information and advice is planned and causes no disruption to treatment.

Often another healthcare worker is present with the patient during the consultation, and the involvement of two healthcare professionals modifies the one-to-one patient–carer relationship found in conventional consultation. We consider the impact of this change in Section 2.3.

Considerable preparation is needed to extract the maximum benefit from the teleconsultation process. Tachakra and Haig [45] identify the following prerequisites:

- *Agree on the purpose of the teleconsultation.* For example, is the session to diagnose a condition, to monitor the progress of treatment or to develop the skills of healthcare workers?

- *Establish the process and content of the teleconsultation.* Whatever its main purpose, the consultation should focus in a natural and continuous way on the relevant healthcare issues. It should avoid irrelevancies and discontinuities as well as distractions such as the need to adjust technology settings.
- *Ensure practitioners are trained in the use of equipment.* To obtain the naturalness mentioned above, practitioners should be familiar with the equipment and its operation.
- *Formalise the delegation of clinical responsibilities.* A doctor who participates in a teleconsultation must be satisfied that any healthcare worker who accompanies the patient at the other end of the link can carry out any medical procedures that are needed.
- *Decide on documentation.* All healthcare professionals involved in the teleconsultation should document the procedure and the outcomes and make sure that a suitable note is made in the patient's medical record.

This is quite a formidable list of requirements and there is merit in developing guidelines and protocols to disseminate good practice and increase efficiency [46] (see Section 2.3.2).

2.2.2   Tele-education

Online information sources, often available over the Internet, are now commonplace. These sources can offer excellent educational material with the benefits of low cost and easy access at the desktop. Where the information is oriented towards medicine or healthcare it fits into our definition of telemedicine in Section 1.2.4. We refer to the use of telemedical links to deliver educational material in this way as *tele-education*.

We can distinguish several types of tele-education depending on who is the recipient and what is the purpose of the transmission:

- clinical education from teleconsultation;
- clinical education via the Internet;
- academic study via the Internet;
- public education via the Internet.

Noting the role of the Internet, we will look at these categories in turn.

Clinical Education from Teleconsultation

Wherever teleconsultation takes place involving a healthcare worker, e.g. a GP or a nurse, and an expert consultant, there is an opportunity for education to occur.

In normal telemedicine practice, the non-expert health carer is in the same room as the patient and the expert consultant is at the other end of the remote link. The non-expert can therefore help the patient to articulate and interpret his or her symptoms and so make it easier for the consultant to give an expert opinion. The non-expert can similarly interpret an expert's diagnosis and recommendations for treatment and reassure the patient.

The non-expert will of course have some general knowledge of the patient's condition. However, by being present during the consultation the non-expert can receive some of the detailed, expert knowledge offered by the consultant and add to his or her knowledge and skills. The education and training are further enhanced by the interactive, intermediary role taken by the generalist compared with passive reading or attendance at a lecture. This is an opportunity not presented by the normal referral process in which the patient sees the GP in the primary care surgery and is referred to the consultant in the acute hospital.

A teledermatology project [47] for patients in rural Wales provides a good example of clinical tele-education carried out in this way.

Clinical Education via the Internet

There are many other examples of clinical tele-education offering variations on the consultation theme described above. More recent instances demonstrate a preference for the Internet and the World Wide Web, making use of their penetration and convenience. Applications range from teleconsultations involving mainly consultant–consultant interaction, through training in rural public health, to virtual conferences and continuing medical education.

Conveniently, several examples are gathered together in one source, the e-health report [6] written by John Mitchell for the Australian government. The author illustrates the applications as case studies, and, although many of them are Australian in origin, they show clearly the range of use and the benefits of tele-education for isolated, rural communities. Table 2.1 summarises a few of the applications.

Together with teleconsultation and the lifelong health record, continuing medical education (CME), i.e. lifelong learning for clinicians, and personalised health education for the public are major themes in Malaysia's Telemedicine Flagship Application described in Section 1.4.2 and elsewhere [39].

While CME can be experienced by taking a formal course, healthcare workers can obviously update and extend their knowledge on a personal basis. Clinicians have specialised access to some excellent web and other online resources which are ideal for this purpose. Examples include national sites such as the UK's National Electronic Library for Health (NELH) [52], the USA's National Library of Medicine (NLM) [53] and the various Cochrane evidence-based medicine sites [54]. Here, they can use specialised databases or literature searching tools such as MEDLINE to retrieve evidence-based information from which to enhance their own skills and the treatment of their patients.

Table 2.1.   Clinical tele-education applications via the Internet [6]

Participants	Application	Reference
Consultants	Teleconsultation/renal videoconferencing	[48]
Surgeons	Virtual conference on surgery	[49]
Health professionals	Online clinical audit	[50]
Clinicians, nurses	Continuing medical education (CME)	[51]

Academic Study via the Internet

Education and training in the traditional sense of organised courses leading to recognised qualifications are also well served by tele-education [55]. Increasingly, universities are offering degree and other courses by distance learning. Most of these telemedical courses are at the postgraduate level and are part of CME.

Collaboration between universities and clinicians in healthcare organisations is also leading to innovative educational programmes. Thus, the non-profit organisation EuroTransMed (ETM) offers programmes by doctors for doctors delivered as weekly interactive broadcasts on chosen medical topics [56]. In a different vein, the Advanced Informatics in Medicine (AIM) project (Section 1.4.3) has developed a resource of units and worked examples for many topics in health informatics, known as IT-EDUCTRA [57, 58]. The units are written by experts and published on the web for course developers to take, modify and use as they wish.

In summary, the future for tele-education for healthcare professionals looks bright. Distance learning via the web is in its infancy and we have yet to understand fully how to use it to 'add value' to conventional text-based courses. Also, the web cannot yet offer the real-time, broadband facilities of videoconferencing and is better suited to publishing and literature searching [59]. However, there is plenty of scope for interaction and creativity, and for making access more extensive and equitable.

Public Education via Telemedicine

Another example of tele-education, also entitled to the description of *tele-information*, concerns education of the community at large about matters of public health. Examples include issues of diet, exercise and hygiene, and information on specific diseases and conditions, such as cancer. The information can be presented (pushed) in a controlled way to a target audience via a kiosk in a shopping mall, health centre or home, or received (pulled) in a less structured way by anyone 'surfing' the web. The same mechanisms can be used to advertise facilities such as surgery hours, pharmacist opening times and so on [60].

As the word 'controlled' implies, the authors of material delivered by the push approach know their audience and design targeted information following discussion with the public. The style and content of the web site can be tailored to the audience and its typical level of knowledge and understanding, e.g. sufferers of a particular disease [61], and carefully evaluated for appropriateness. The web pages can inform readers and answer frequently asked questions (FAQs), as well as act as a clearing house for email communication and chat lines so that people with common interests and concerns can gain support from others. This community self-support aspect is a powerful feature of such sites [62].

The great merit of push sites is that they are not only comprehensive but also at the right level to educate and inform. In contrast, most of the information on the web is unregulated and presented for a specialist audience. Although usually reliable—the source will indicate the credentials—it is seldom validated and it may be too technical or designed for a more sophisticated audience than has access to it (see Section 6.4). Either way, the information can be difficult for a layperson to digest or appraise critically and may present a case of 'a little learning is a dangerous thing'.

Information may also be incomplete, e.g. costs may be omitted or complicating pathologies ignored. These omissions increase the risk to the patient or their relatives if the information is taken at face value, and the frustration to the physician, who has to explain its unsuitability. Problems can also arise from out-of-date or absent hyperlinks which produce spurious or no information.

The Internet user must be aware of these potential pitfalls. In general, however, the benefits of a more informed public increasingly involved in, and able to take responsibility for, their own care easily outweigh the possible problems. The web certainly has the ability to change the doctor–patient relationship for the good as well as for the bad (see Sections 2.3.3 and 6.4).

We should remember, however, that radio and television offer well-tried alternatives for public health education that reach much greater audiences than the Internet [63].

2.2.3   Telemonitoring

Telemonitoring is the use of a telecommunications link to gather routine or repeated data on a patient's condition. The acquisition process may be manual, in which case the patient records the data and transmits them by telephone, facsimile or a computer/modem system. Alternatively, the acquisition may be entirely automated so that continuous data can be submitted either in real time or in store-and-forward mode.

The patient may be in a hospital, at home, on an aircraft or wearing an ambulatory device [64] such as a blood pressure monitor, and data can be transmitted across the world. In almost every case, the purpose of monitoring is to decide if and when an adjustment is needed to the patient's treatment. The adjustment can be communicated verbally by telephone or automatically using a touch-tone telephone and a computer telephone integrated (CTI) system. Randomised trials have shown the approach to improve the condition of home-based patients with hypertension [65] and diabetes [66].

An interesting variation on the CTI approach is to issue automatic reminders to patients at home to take their medication at the pre-set time. Forgetting to take prescribed medication is a significant cause of instability in the condition of many patients.

The above cases are largely those in which the monitored conditions are unlikely to become critical over a short period. However, telemonitoring is also successful in potentially life-threatening circumstances such as heart conditions (telecardiology). Examples include ECGs routed from elderly patients at home to their GPs [67] and ultrasound scans transmitted from new-born infants to paediatric cardiologists [68].

As several of the examples suggest, however, telemonitoring is likely to find increasing application in telecare, particularly for elderly and disabled people confined to their own homes or institutions. Increased use for unwell travellers is also anticipated.

2.2.4   Telesurgery

Compared with the other 'tele' applications discussed so far, *telesurgery* is in its infancy [69, 70]. It is practised in two ways. Telementoring, as we have seen (Section 1.4.2 and [29]), describes the assistance given by specialists to surgeons carrying out a surgical procedure at a remote location. Typically, the assistance is offered via a video and audio connection that can extend elsewhere in the building or over a satellite link to another country.[1] Clearly, there is a strong element of tele-education in telementoring.

The other approach is *telepresence surgery*, which guides robotic arms to carry out remote surgical procedures. In this case, the term 'remote' may describe comparatively short distances as well as large ones since the surgeon manipulates interfaces connected mechanically and electronically to surgical instruments such as scalpels and needles. The links allow large movements of the surgeon's hands to be scaled down so that very precise, tremor-free incisions can be made. The technique, known as *movement scaling*, has the potential to allow doctors to repair damage inside vessels [69].

2.3   PATIENTS AND CARERS

All of the different types of telemedicine described in Section 2.2 involve the patient and carers in some way or other. But how do telemedicine and telecare influence the patient's experience compared with other, conventional,

---

[1]   The author once sat in a lecture theatre in Montreal and watched a live telecast of surgeons removing a patient's gallstones in Strasbourg.

approaches? What makes a teleconsultation or tele-education different from a conventional consultation or information gathering? Are these differences critical and how should we deal with them? What preparation and organisation are needed to conduct a successful teleconsultation? We will explore some of these issues under the following headings:

- patient perceptions;
- carers and procedures;
- the changing knowledge base.

Note that we are concerned here with the way telemedicine affects the participants. We look at the development, organisation and delivery of telemedicine services in Chapter 5, where we pick up patients' expectations of telemedicine services.

2.3.1   Patient Perceptions

Stanberry [11] quotes the results of a study by Tachakra *et al.* [71] of attitudes of patients new to teleconsultation. The patients were concerned over their privacy and the confidentiality of information, including others overhearing the conversation in the teleconsultation environment (50%), videotaping of the proceedings (56%) and the subsequent use of videotapes for teaching purposes (65%).

Barring exceptional circumstances of public interest [27], patients have a right to expect that their health conditions are treated with absolute confidentiality according to standard medical ethics [72]. Because telemedicine is new, however, it is quite common for non-clinical persons to ask if they can observe a teleconsultation session. It is therefore essential that these persons are introduced to the patient over the link and that he or she is asked to grant permission for the visitors to remain. Only in this way can the patient's perception and expectation of confidentiality be assured. We return to the legal and security issues of telemedicine in Section 2.5 and in Chapter 6.

Although confidentiality was identified as a concern in the Tachakra survey, the study found that patients were even more fearful about the clinical risk presented by the new technology: 94% were afraid that the television monitor would not display the medical condition with sufficient clarity to allow accurate diagnosis or treatment, and more than 79% felt that doctors would avoid malpractice litigation by blaming the technology or editing the video transcriptions.

Some of these criticisms can be put down to nervousness associated with any unfamiliar process and, indeed, patients express less concern after repeated experience of telemedicine.

However, the concerns about doctors' avoidance of litigation demonstrate a want of trust on the part of patients. The healthcare system may provide the background for this suspicion (as in litigious USA) but its more direct cause is the impersonal nature of the technology, which can intrude between the patient and the carer. The patient perceives the technology as a refuge within which physicians can hide and patients have little redress. Where necessary, therefore, telemedicine practitioners have a duty to ensure that patients are properly informed of their rights under the law before they participate in teleconsultations.

Most teleconsultations take place in a doctor's surgery or in a hospital setting. However, an interesting effect arises in telecare where teleconsultations take place with patients confined to their own homes without a carer or technician present.

These patients receive training in the use of videoconferencing and other equipment, and they quickly become adept at its deployment. They acquire considerable experience and learn tweaks that they can make to improve the quality of the teleconsultation process. The patients' confidence, and their perceived control and expertise, allows them to focus on their medical condition, giving more accurate descriptions and becoming more involved in their own treatment [32]. This process offers an excellent example of tele-education and the skilling that can accompany the teleconsultation process.[2]

Naturally, the 'expert' telepatient must have the mental and physical capabilities to acquire the necessary knowledge and skills. This may not be possible with elderly patients, particularly those who are mentally confused. Such patients are perhaps the most difficult to treat by telemedicine since they find the process so disturbing. Their distress is heightened by the impersonal nature of the technology [73], which is superficially similar to television but requires them to interact rather than watch passively. In the patient's normal experience only 'real' people ask them questions, not images on a television screen, and they have difficulty in locating the source of the query.

2.3.2 Carers and Procedures

The patient's perception of teleconsultation is intimately linked with the treatment he or she receives. We have already commented (Sections 2.2.1 and 2.2.2) upon the change that telemedicine brings to the consultation process by involving another healthcare professional situated with the patient in the clinical examination or interview. This person can act as an intermediary

---

[2] On a visit to the Queen Elizabeth Hospital in Adelaide, the author once sat in on a routine videoconferencing link involving a renal dialysis patient in the Australian outback. It was impressive to see the ease with which the patient participated, even to the point of remonstrating with the 'experts' at the hospital end of the link to position the video camera correctly and not to move too much or too quickly. Interestingly, the healthcare workers took great pains to introduce the author to the patient, explaining who he was and why he was there, and asking her if she was happy that he participated in the session.

between the patient and the consultant, helping both parties to interpret the other's questions and statements.

The advocacy offered by the second healthcare worker can be immensely helpful and reassuring to the patient daunted by personal medical concerns, the medical jargon, and, if that is not enough, the technology. This support role is not necessarily a part of the healthcare worker's normal activity, however, and some prior training may be needed to develop the interpersonal skills to discharge it effectively.

It is also vital that the consultant is satisfied that the healthcare professional with the patient is competent to carry out any treatment that is delegated to him or her [45, 74], including those procedures that cannot be carried out in the teleconsultation itself or are left to later. This requirement includes the ability to capture the information needed for treatment—a competence that should be confirmed before the teleconsultation begins.

It may well be useful for other healthcare workers to be present at the consultation so that they can acquire the skills for future participation. These training sessions should be documented carefully to determine the skill levels and evaluation procedures of all involved.

One interesting consequence of such local skilling (tele-education) is that it may make the telemedicine link redundant.

In describing the essential features of teleconsultation (Section 2.2.1) we noted Tachakra and Haig's [45] prerequisites for success. Where there are frequent changes of healthcare personnel it can be helpful to document the teleconsultation procedure by providing either a *process guideline* or template of the steps involved, or a protocol or pathway for the medical treatment [45].

A process guideline consists of a detailed checklist that might include the following stages:

- explain the purpose and process to the patient;
- establish the remote link;
- introduce the participants;
- summarise the patient's condition and purpose of the session;
- review the patient's history;
- perform the examination or interview;
- review other evidence such as test results;
- discuss diagnosis;
- discuss prognosis and management of the condition;
- address any other concerns or queries;
- close the remote link and the session.

Tachakra and Haig explain these stages in more detail but the sequence and purpose are evident from this simple checklist. The list ensures that no essentials are omitted and that all participants are working to achieve the same outcomes.

Alongside the process guideline, healthcare professionals may choose to establish an integrated care pathway (ICP) [75, 76] documenting the patient's care and including the teleconsultation as an integral part of the care process. ICPs are outside the scope of this book but we can summarise the main benefits [75, 77].

- *Improved patient outcomes*: the multidisciplinary nature of ICPs, plus the emphasis on outcomes and tracking variances from expectations, leads to a review process directed to improving outcomes.
- *Improved teamwork*: the multidisciplinary approach gives carers a better understanding of the holistic nature of the care process and their roles within it.
- *Improved consistency*: the aim is to devise ICPs that lay down a generalised standard of care.
- *Increased patient involvement*: the documented pathway follows the patient through the care process. It therefore offers them a fuller understanding of their treatment and progress.
- *Continuous audit*: variance tracking provides the raw material for continuous clinical audit as well as iterative improvement of the ICP itself.
- *Resource management and contracting*: a carefully constructed ICP can ensure that clinical tests and drugs are deployed only when they are needed and can maximise benefit.
- *Risk management*: ICPs offer the opportunity to anticipate and control risk.

Each of these benefits may lead to changes in the teleconsultation process and its guideline, and improvements in patient care [78].

An interesting study by Randles has also examined at length the effect of telecommunication links on physician–physician interactions in the absence of patients [79]. The results allowed the researchers to construct a model of medical decision support based on the diagnostic process and type of teleconsultation provided. The model explains how telemedicine fosters support and teamwork among physicians and offers guidance on the development and operation of telemedicine programmes.

2.3.3   The Changing Knowledge Base

This part of our discussion relates back to the review of tele-education presented in Section 2.2.2. There we investigated the education and skilling of patients and carers via teleconsultations and the Internet in some detail and we need not repeat that process here. What we must do here, however, is draw out some of the consequences of the changing knowledge base between carers and patients.

Patients are becoming more knowledgeable about medical advances, their choices and their rights. Frequently, the informed patient knows more about his or her (sometimes supposed) condition than the GP, who does not have the time to surf the Internet and dredge up the latest information on the most obscure ailments.

This is a problem not only for the GP but also for the patient, who is badly in need of advice on how to assess the mound of data and make use of it. But the GP lacks the training to find out what the patient needs let alone how to supply it. For a long time, the very essence of clinical education has been the notion that the clinician is the expert and the patient is a layperson who lacks the ability to understand a medical explanation even if it were given to him or her. So why bother?

This dilemma is amply illustrated by a perceptive editorial that appeared in the *British Medical Journal* [80] pointing out that patients want more than simply information about their conditions; they want involvement too.

2.4   BENEFITS AND LIMITATIONS OF TELEMEDICINE

Our journey through the origins, development and drivers of telemedicine, and our categorisation of the various types, has revealed many of the benefits and limitations. Our purpose here, therefore, is to summarise these factors in one convenient place and to say a little more about some of them. When considering the limitations we concentrate on clinical and operational factors, leaving external constraints such as technical and legal issues to Section 2.5.

2.4.1   Benefits of Telemedicine

We can summarise the principal benefits claimed for telemedicine as follows:

- better access to healthcare;
- access to better healthcare;
- improved communication between carers;
- easier and better continuing education;
- better access to information;
- better resource utilisation;
- reduced costs.

These benefits are clearly interrelated but we can deal with them in turn, building on comments made in previous sections.

Better Access to Healthcare

Extending healthcare access to rural communities and disadvantaged populations, poorly served or without these facilities, is still one of the major drivers of telemedicine (Section 1.4.2). This socio-economic impetus has provided a strategic aspect to telemedicine programmes in several countries [81, 82].

Greater convenience to patients by reducing travel and disruption is also a benefit sought for and claimed by the majority of projects. Time savings for both patient and carer and faster access to care are similarly easy to demonstrate where they occur. Telecare offers many examples of these benefits.

Access to Better Healthcare

Any healthcare is obviously better where none existed before (see above) but under this heading we are looking for improvements in the quality of care. A clear benefit of telemedicine is the remote access that a patient and his or her physician have to specialist advice when it is not available locally.

Early intervention, more seamless care (including care protocols) and better monitoring of progress [83] are additional advantages of telemedicine links involving a primary care doctor [73], a hospital specialist and a community care nurse. As we have seen, the monitoring process may also entail tele-monitoring (Section 2.2.3).

Improved Communication between Carers

The shift to digital information offers numerous benefits for carers and their patients. Digitised data such as a patient's previous history, X-rays, test results and notes for the current episode are readily transmitted electronically using standard protocols and technologies such as email [73]. Discharge letters are similarly available without delay.

Digital communication provides healthcare information that is more accurate, more complete and more timely—attributes of quality that lead to better access and better healthcare.

Easier and Better Continuing Education

The discussion on tele-education (Section 2.2.2) dealt with this issue at length and we need add little here. One scenario not mentioned in the literature is worth a passing thought, namely the provision of healthcare courses, perhaps with awards, for the general public.

Several countries are promoting a subsidised scheme for low-income families to help them gain home access to the Internet. Low-income groups are often those identified as being at greatest risk from disease due to socio-economic conditions and lifestyle. The Internet could be used for health promotion with web sites targeting both children and parents. It could also be used to advertise health programmes such as cervical smear campaigns and facilities such as local fitness centres. Incentives could be provided to encourage take-up. The opportunities are endless.

Better Access to Information

The continuing education benefit referred to under the last heading is an example of the 'push' technology outlined in Section 2.2.2. Better access to information is concerned more with the individual endeavouring to 'pull' information from the Internet and/or other sources to answer specific questions.

The individual mentioned here may be a doctor accessing 'case-oriented' information in an electronic library [73], accessing the literature with an electronic search engine, or visiting a web site to find out about events of interest or the latest medical equipment [84]. Alternatively, he or she may be a patient wanting information on a medical condition, times of surgery hours, or advice on how to stop smoking. It's all out there somewhere!

Better Resource Utilisation

Better access to healthcare and access to better healthcare are one side of the access coin. Better resource utilisation is the other side. It is uneconomic to replicate resources in several centres when these resources have infrequent use. A preferred approach is therefore to set up a smaller number of resource sites and make these available to potential users via telemedical links.

The arrangement can apply to the disposition of both specialist and expensive equipment such as MRI machines as well as to 'walk-in' centres for patients with minor complaints [85]. Any spare capacity in the telemedicine network can be used for a range of tele-education purposes.

Reduced Costs

This is the most contentious benefit since few protagonists of telemedicine have been able to show cost savings in an unequivocal way. One of the reasons is that telemedicine trials often involve few presenting patients and it is not clear how costs and benefits scale.

Clear cost savings have been demonstrated in teleradiology, which has been around long enough for practitioners to create a marketable service and optimise its operation [35]. There is also evidence for economic benefits from telemedicine in home healthcare [86] and the care of prison inmates [87]. We give the cost–benefit issue fuller study in Chapter 5.

2.4.2   Limitations of Telemedicine

Our survey of the reported limitations of telemedicine includes the following:

- poor patient–carer relationships;
- poor relationships between healthcare professionals;
- impersonal technology;
- organisational disruption;

- additional training needs;
- difficult protocol development;
- uncertain quality of health information;
- low rates of utilisation.

Poor Patient–Carer Relationships

The intrusion of technology between the patient and the carer is a potential source of contention, particularly if the electronic devices require constant adjustment or they breakdown. On the other hand, we have also pointed out the enhancement of the patient–carer relationship when a second healthcare worker is involved. Poorer relationships are therefore by no means automatic and are often confined to the start-up stage of a link.

Patient concerns about the suitability of the equipment and the confidentiality of the consultation have also been mentioned, as have the reservations of both patient and physician about the possibilities of litigation (Section 2.3.1). These fears will take more time to overcome [73, 88].

Poor Relationships between Healthcare Professionals

Telemedicine can represent a threat to status and preferred practices. The likelihood of such threats is enhanced if one of more of the clinical participants is over-enthusiastic and tries to coerce unconvinced colleagues into using the link without due discussion or preparation.

An interesting paper [89] with the title 'How not to develop telemedicine systems' gives good advice on avoiding this trap (see also [90, 91]). Most of the errors identified fall into the 'technology' or 'bureaucracy driven' category, so leaving insufficient emphasis on the clinical benefits.

Impersonal Technology

We need add little to our previous discussion (Section 2.3.1) except to reiterate that the problems are most likely to occur with technophobic patients (or healthcare workers). Their incidence is therefore greatest with elderly patients whose lack of confidence fuels their confusion. Careful preparation and equipment maintenance will minimise most difficulties.

Organisational Disruption

The introduction of new technologies and methods of working always lead to some disruption and concern about the short- and long-term consequences. The US Western Governors' Association Telemedicine Action Report [73, 92] lists several reasons for resisting change, including:

- fear that telemedicine will increase the workload;
- fear that telemedicine is market- rather than user-driven;

- fear of technological obsolescence;
- lack of skills and the need to acquire them;
- lack of agreed standards.

These concerns all represent clinical risks and should be included in risk assessment at the time of considering a proposal for a telemedicine service (see Section 5.4.4).

Additional Training Needs

Education and training are key elements but considerable overheads in a successful telemedicine application. Both start-up and ongoing requirements must be considered as the system develops and new staff are taken on board. The educational need is directed towards alerting clinicians of the potential of telemedicine and convincing sceptics of its value [91]. The seasoned enthusiast will demonstrate to these sceptics 'what's in it for them'.

The training requirement covers [91] the setting up and use of the equipment, the teleconsultation process, and the production of appropriate documentation for these tasks and for recording the consultation procedures and outcomes.

Difficult Protocol Development

Protocol or pathway development is one of the most important and most time-consuming aspects of the introduction of a telemedicine application. The value of a care pathway is premised on the basis of multidisciplinary involvement; a requirement which is both the strength and the Achilles' heel of the approach [77]. The strength comes from the holistic and integrated view of care that arises from multidisciplinary team working. The weakness follows from the unequal status of the participants (e.g. doctors and nurses) and the shear logistical difficulties of getting staff together to work on and agree the pathway.

The very process of protocol and pathways development may also turn up hidden resource requirements. The development should therefore be seen as an advantage in that it identifies and costs what is needed to run a telemedical service properly. Too often, however, the protocol will be seen as a nuisance by telemedicine enthusiasts and a weapon by sceptics.

Uncertain Quality of Health Information

We have covered this aspect in Section 2.2.2 on tele-education, where we echoed concerns over the unregulated nature of much of the information on the web.

Nancy Brown from the government-funded US Telemedicine Information Exchange [93] adds a valuable chapter [94] to Wootton and Craig's book that directs users to the best Internet sources for information on telemedicine and telecare.

Low Rates of Utilisation

We offered 'improved rates of utilisation' as an advantage in the previous section. But what if a telemedical link is installed in enthusiasm and then remains unused, or the link is so successful that local healthcare workers become so proficient that they make the links redundant?

Fortunately, as we shall see (Chapter 3), most telemedicine equipment is relatively inexpensive and sufficiently flexible [21] that it can be used for a pilot study or pressed into service elsewhere within the organisation.

2.5   BARRIERS TO PROGRESS

Whereas the previous section dealt with some operational limitations of telemedicine, this one addresses factors external to telemedical practice that will nevertheless inhibit its development unless they are either removed or clarified. Several of the barriers we consider arise from the ways in which the remote link between the carer and the patient changes how healthcare professionals work and assume responsibility for care.

Tanriverdi and Iacona [95] have considered the reasons why the diffusion of telemedicine is limited and the number of teleconsultations is small compared with conventional consultations. They suggest that knowledge barriers have to be overcome in several areas before take-up is possible, and classify these barriers as technical, economic, organisational and behavioural. Our list of barriers focuses on specific issues in the following categories:

- telecommunications infrastructure and standards;
- cost effectiveness;
- national policy and strategy;
- ethical and legal aspects.

All of these factors arise naturally within the context of issues we discuss in subsequent chapters. For example, we devote a complete chapter (Chapter 6) to ethical and legal issues. At this stage, therefore, we simply outline the constraints these factors can impose on telemedicine practice and development, leaving detailed discussion to later.

Telecommunications Infrastructure and Standards

For telemedicine to work there must be a telecommunications link between a patient and a remote carer. This link is usually a physical connection although increasingly it is a wireless circuit (see Section 3.4.5). Most links between, rather than within, buildings are multipurpose, i.e. they are installed as general electronic highways to handle many different services. A potential barrier to the practice of telemedicine is therefore the bandwidth [21] of the shared link, i.e. its capacity to carry telemedical data.

The bandwidth will be low if it is based on analogue rather than digital transmission or, if it is digital, shared with many other users, as is the Internet. These circumstances will limit the type of information that can be transmitted. For example, it may not be possible to transfer large images such as X-rays or even to establish usable videoconferencing links.

Another technical factor that can lead to difficulty is the incompatibility of operating standards or protocols [96], especially across international boundaries, so that transmitted data are either not received or are unintelligible to the receiving station.

The technical aspects of telemedicine are considered in detail in Chapter 3. Our purpose here is to point out that restricted bandwidth and poor adherence to interoperability standards can be significant barriers to progress in telemedicine.

Cost Effectiveness

The cost effectiveness of telemedicine is a major subject of debate within the telemedicine community and we give it due attention in Chapter 5. There are two main reasons for the debate. The first is that the majority of pilot studies were (and still are) funded by government and academic grants, and they have been more concerned with technical and clinical feasibility than cost effectiveness.

The second is that it is actually quite difficult to evaluate the cost benefits of a telemedicine application [97]. As we saw above, a telemedicine system may be used for other purposes and it may be difficult to apportion charges. Also, it is often hard to cost advantages such as increased convenience, higher quality, more equitable access and so on. Again, public and private regulation and payment may prevent the full realisation of service and income generation opportunities.

Telemedicine advocates are now trying to address these difficulties [35, 97, 98] but the uncertain cost benefits have deterred commercial companies from entering the field. Unless these studies find ways to demonstrate cost effectiveness, the uncertainty will remain a major barrier to progress.

National Policy and Strategy

In Section 1.4.2 we identified health policy as a driver of telemedicine, so how come we now brand it as a barrier? The answer is simple—if a factor is a driver for progress then its absence can act as a brake. We said so in Section 1.6.

Certain countries, e.g. the USA [3, 19], Australia [4, 6] and, most notably, Malaysia [38, 39], have realised the importance of healthcare planning involving telemedicine and have begun to evolve policies and enact laws that encourage its development. Other countries, e.g. the UK [36, 37], have adopted a more 'bottom-up' approach, issuing guidelines and advice but avoiding direction.

It is possible that these different approaches reflect the perceived value and applicability of telemedicine within a country. However, there is no doubt that the coordinated action of the planners will produce more rapid and successful development than the fragmented stance taken within the UK. We tease out these arguments in Chapter 5.

Ethical and Legal Aspects

As indicated at the start of this section, we have a whole chapter dedicated to ethics and the legal aspects of telemedicine in Chapter 6. It is nevertheless useful to summarise here some of the conundrums that present themselves to clinicians and healthcare managers concerned with offering and operating telemedicine services.

We list the key issues [11] that we address later to show the range of concerns:

- confidentiality and security;
- patients' right of access;
- data protection;
- duty of care;
- standards of care;
- malpractice;
- suitability and failure of equipment;
- physician licensure and accreditation;
- physician reimbursement;
- intellectual property rights.

That is a daunting list! Interestingly, all of the items in the list apply to conventional medicine but the 'at-a-distance' aspect of telemedicine, the dependence on telecommunications equipment, and the technical, but non-clinical, expertise to operate it raise new questions.

Let us consider just three examples to illustrate the point.

- If a patient resident in a city has access to a treatment, then does a patient with a similar condition living in a remote community have a right to similar treatment if it can be facilitated by a telemedicine link?
- Is a consultant physician trained and licensed to practice medicine in one country able to give advice across a telemedicine link to colleagues in another country? What are the consequences if as a result of this advice a patient suffers harm?

• How is a physician not employed by a healthcare organisation reimbursed for his or her expert advice offered over a telemedical link?

We need guidelines and answers to these questions and new ones that arise as we learn more about remote medicine. Without them the benefits of telemedicine and telecare will not be realised to their full extent.

2.6 SUMMARY

In Chapter 2 we have seen that:

• Currently, there are four different types of telemedicine: teleconsultation, tele-education, telemonitoring and telesurgery.
• Patient perceptions of telemedicine show that they are concerned about confidentiality and, more importantly, about the clinical risks of the new technology and the possibility that clinicians will blame the system to avoid litigation.
• The advocacy offered by a second healthcare worker in a teleconsultation can be helpful and reassuring to the patient.
• It can be helpful to document the teleconsultation procedure by providing either a guideline or template of the steps involved, or a protocol or pathway for the medical treatment.
• Patients are becoming more knowledgeable about medical advances, their choices and their rights. This is a problem not only for the GP but also for the patient, who is badly in need of advice on how to assess the mound of data and make use of it.
• The benefits of telemedicine include better access to healthcare, access to better healthcare, improved communication between carers, easier and better continuing education, better access to information, better resource utilisation and reduced costs.
• The limitations of telemedicine include poor patient-carer relationships and relationships between healthcare professionals, impersonal technology, organisational disruption, additional training needs, difficult protocol development, uncertain quality of health information, and low rates of utilisation.
• The barriers to progress of telemedicine include telecommunications infrastructure and standards, cost effectiveness, national policy and strategy, and ethical and legal aspects.

3
TECHNOLOGY OF TELEMEDICINE SYSTEMS

OBJECTIVES

At the end of this chapter you should be able to:

- distinguish the types of information used in telemedicine systems;
- understand the bandwidth, compression and storage requirements of such systems;
- realise the range and importance of standards for information transmission;
- identify the image capture and videoconferencing components of telemedicine systems;
- recognise the telemonitoring devices used by telemedicine specialists;
- consider the telecommunications options available for telemedicine installations;
- discuss the system integration needs of telemedicine links.

3.1 INTRODUCTION

In this chapter we take a look at the technology needed to set up and operate a telemedicine service. We consider the service providers and applications in Chapter 4 and the strategic and business issues in Chapter 5. We also assume that the main purpose of the service is teleconsultation, including some telemonitoring with medical peripherals.

This chapter begins by identifying the types of information we want to use in our service since the data transfer requirements will determine the nature and cost of the equipment we use. We also discuss how we can improve performance using data compression techniques.

With a knowledge of information types we review the elements of a typical telemedicine system to see how we capture, transmit and display information. This survey then leads to a consideration of the telecommunication options for constructing the remote link between the transmitting and receiving stations, including the current 'hot topic', wireless systems.

At this stage we have a good idea of the technology requirements of our new telemedicine service and so finally we look briefly at some of the operational and integration issues surrounding the introduction of the new technology.

3.2   INFORMATION TYPES AND TRANSMISSION

3.2.1   Types of Telemedicine Information

In a face-to-face consultation, a physician might use some combination of all five senses—sight, sound, touch, smell and taste—to assess a patient's condition. The first three methods are by far the most common (thankfully!) and the sensory data are transmitted directly from the patient to the observer.

In telemedicine, however, the sensory data are first converted into electrical impulses for transmission to the remote physician. Methods to convert smell and taste stimuli into electrical signals are still in the experimental stage and, while the sense of touch can be translated successfully into an electrical equivalent, the reverse process is more difficult and not well understood. Hence, a teleconsultation relies primarily on the two senses of sight and sound. The information (useful data) derived from these senses can be divided into four types:

- text and data;
- audio;
- still (single) images;
- video (sequential images).

Table 3.1 gives telemedicine examples of these types along with their typical file size in kilo- or megabytes following digitisation.

The wide range of electronic files sizes from these sources suggests the need to match the choice and performance characteristics of the telemedicine equipment to the clinical need. Under- and over-specification of systems can otherwise lead to disappointment and premature abandonment of a promising project.

Table 3.1.   Typical examples of telemedicine information (after Falconer [21])

Source	Type	Typical file size
Patient notes	Text	< 10 KB
Electronic stethoscope	Audio	100 KB
Chest X-ray	Still image	1 MB
Foetal ultrasound (30 s)	Video	10 MB

Let us look at the relevant features of these information types in more detail.

3.2.2   Text and Data

Electronic documents such as reports, correspondence or medical records containing ASCII or Unicode text and numerical information can be transmitted directly in digital format. The digitised file can be edited with a word processor, database or spreadsheet program but this is seldom necessary, or even desirable, since the transmitted information is invariably 'read-only'.

If a document is only available in paper format then it can be digitised for transmission with either a scanner (e.g. fax) or a document camera. Unless the text is subjected to optical character recognition (OCR) [99] it will be in bitmapped format and cannot be edited.

Frequently, textual information is needed before the teleconsultation takes place or later, as a consequence of the process. In these cases it is more efficient to send the documents by post or, better still, as attachments to emails (Section 3.5.2).

3.2.3   Audio

The *public switched telephone network* (PSTN but sometimes known as the plain old telephone system, POTS) can be used to transmit sound (e.g. speech) and establish a remote diagnosis. However, the quality (ease of understanding) and bandwidth (capacity to carry information) of analogue telephony are seldom adequate for medical applications. In contrast, digital signals can be transmitted over networks for large distances without degradation. Digital signals can also be manipulated (Section 3.2.6) to improve system performance.

An analogue sound is digitised by sampling its amplitude at discrete time intervals to recreate the waveform. The discrete nature of the digitisation process introduces *quantisation* or amplitude round-off errors as the digital sample value approximates the analogue signal at a given instant. The human ear detects this error as a hissing noise and to reduce the effect the sample value should have a resolution of at least 1 in 65 536 (2^{16}), giving a 16-bit quantisation error.

Special sound cards, e.g. the Creative Labs SoundBlaster card, that slot easily into a PC are available for this purpose and, once installed, no special equipment other than a suitable microphone is needed for teleconsultations. These cards can also receive audio output directly from medical peripherals such as an ultrasound scanner [21]. Under the Windows operating system found on most PCs, audio files are held in a standardised WAV format for easy transmission and reception. Alternative formats are available for other platforms [100].

More specialised sources [101] will tell you about the various encoding techniques used to sample and digitise audio signals and the effects of other parameters such as sampling rate.

3.2.4   Still Images

Still image quality is defined by the size of a *pixel* (picture element) in an image and the number of *grey* or *colour* levels. These parameters are determined by the quality of the scanning device which uses photosensitive, charge coupled diode (CCD) transducers to digitise the image.

The smaller the pixel size, the more pixels there are in a given picture and the higher the resolution of the image. Flat-bed scanning devices [102] typically scan at up to 1200 dots or pixels per inch (dpi) while the new breed of digital cameras [103] can easily produce a 35 mm size transparency image with 1000×1200 pixels, i.e. with a pixel density of over two million.[1]

Each pixel is allocated a fixed number of bits to represent its *grey-scale* level or colour—usually up to 8 bits (255 levels) for grey-scale and up to 24 bits (16.77 million levels) for colour. (depth). The human eye actually fails to detect differences in quality at values far below these levels. However, if the number of bits is too low then both grey-scale and colour images lose resolution and tend to monochrome pictures in which detail is lost in amorphous blocks.

So why not use the maximum number of bits all of the time? The answer is the amount of computer memory or disk space needed to store a high-resolution image, and the bandwidth and time taken to transfer it. For example, The American College of Radiologists (ACR) has defined [104] two categories of teleradiology images; *small matrix* or low-resolution systems must digitise 500 pixel $\times$ 500 pixel $\times$ 8 bit images, while for *large matrix* or high-resolution, systems the required image resolution is 2000 pixel $\times$ 2000 pixel $\times$ 12 bit. A single image file at the low resolution (ultrasound, magnetic resonance, nuclear medicine) standard is therefore about 250 KB. In contrast, a single image file at the high resolution (digitised radiographic films and computed radiography) standard takes 4 MB, a factor of 16 times the small matrix file size.

If a radiologist wanted a full 24-bit (true) colour image of the high matrix image the file size would be 12 MB. Fortunately, radiologists seldom require colour images but teledermatologists do need high resolution and colour depth to show clearly lesions on the skin [105].

In some circumstances, an image can be captured directly by an inexpensive video camera or from the video output of medical devices such as an

---

[1]   Conventional film still packs four million pixels into the same area and it is of much higher resolution since the random dispersion of film pixels compared with the regimented array of the digital image avoids discontinuities in tonal gradations.

ultrasound scanner. The camera signal is then fed to a video capture card in a PC and software used to convert still frames to digital images [21]. If high-resolution images are needed then the equipment becomes much more expensive although prices will inevitably fall.

3.2.5   Video

Our perception of video is conditioned by television to the extent that a videoconference between patient or carer and consultant is regarded as the normal practice of telemedicine. Where video is needed, for example, to demonstrate a patient's mobility after a hip replacement, it is usually sufficient to use a commercial videoconferencing unit (Section 3.3.2) rather than the much more expensive broadcast television. The output from such units approaches broadcast quality.

An important consideration for international teleconsultations is the compatibility of the analogue video signals, and therefore the video equipment, in different countries. There are two widely used formats for analogue video:

- the *National Television Standards Committee* (NTSC) system adopted in North America and Japan, having 525 lines per picture and a frame rate of 30 pictures per second;
- the *Phase Alternating Line* (PAL) system used throughout Western Europe and Australasia, having 625 lines per picture and a frame rate of 25 pictures per second.

France, Russia and the former Warsaw Pact countries have a third system, *Sequential Couleur à Memoire* (SECAM) but this appears to find little use in telemedicine. Most modern television receivers and video recorders are able to convert signals from one standard to another.

The *Common Intermediate Format* (CIF) is a format introduced to provide compatibility between NTSC and PAL and offers a lower resolution of 288 lines per picture at 30 pictures per second. The whole area of video formats and standards is littered with acronyms and obscure terminology, which the interested reader can delve into at reference [106].

3.2.6   Still Image and Video Compression

If still image sizes create problems for image storage and transmission then you can imagine the difficulties presented by video pictures. A CIF video image of 352×288 pixels with an image depth of 24 bits occupies 0.304 Mbytes. At a transmission rate of 25 images per second, the system has therefore to move 7.5 MB per second. Even a quarter-size (QCIF) image of 176×144 pixels requires a rate of 1.9 MB per second.

To reduce these problems and transmission costs, digitised images are therefore compressed in size by hardware or software before transmission and the receiving station then decompresses the transmitted image to display it.

Image compression may be *lossless*, in which case the compression/decompression (*codec*) algorithm is reversible without losing data or the full resolution of the original image. Alternatively, the algorithm can be *lossy*, in which event it discards data to achieve higher compression ratios and decompression cannot recover the original image with its full definition. Lossless compression ratios are typically 1.5–3 : 1 whereas the lossy equivalent may reach ratios of 20 or even 100 : 1. Except in some radiology applications, lossy compression is usually acceptable for telemedicine work.

The lossy compression standard for still images is the *Joint Photographic Expert Group* (JPEG). JPEG can operate on any number of colours. For digital video files a JPEG compression ratio of 100 : 1 may still not be enough. Thus, to push the QCIF image in the previous example down an ISDN-2 line (Section 3.4.3) operating at 128 kilobits per second (Kbps) demands a compression ratio of nearly 120 : 1.

A different codec known as the *Moving Picture Expert Group* (MPEG) is therefore used for video images. MPEG uses a form of *frame differencing* or *motion prediction* based on the assumption that only small parts of a video image change from one frame to the next. If this is so, then a frame sequence can be recaptured by storing the differences between successive frames and adding these to a decompressed base image. The base image is updated with a new fully compressed 'key' frame from time to time to preserve quality, especially with images that contain a lot of rapid motion. MPEG is an asymmetric codec, taking longer to compress the image, so that decompression is more efficient and faster.

There are several alternatives to JPEG and MPEG [107], including some developed especially for radiology work [104]. Table 3.2 gives some examples of typical telemedicine data and compression ratios (see Della Mea [108]).

3.2.7   Frame Rate and Bandwidth

Video frame rates of 25 discrete pictures per second and above fool the human brain into perceiving continuous and smooth motion. However, when video compression takes place, the display frame rate may fall due to the time needed to decompress the images. The effective frame rate may drop to 7.5, 10 or 15 frames per second.

At the lower rates, the sequence of events on screen appears discontinuous and jerky, an effect known as *motion artefact*, which can be disconcerting to patients as well as to carers, all of whom are concerned at the consequences of missing vital information related to diagnosis and treatment.

The ultimate solution to this problem is of course to increase the bandwidth at a cost. A no-cost, sometimes acceptable compromise is to reduce the size of

Table 3.2.   Typical telemedicine data and compression ratios (see Della Mea [108])

Data type	Single image size	Uncompressed file size (MB)	Compressed file size (KB)	Compression ratio
Radiograph	$2000 \times 2000 \times 12$	5.7	285	20 : 1
Pathology microscope image	$800 \times 600 \times 24$	1.44	96	15 : 1
Dermatology image	$1280 \times 1024 \times 24$	3.9	980	4 : 1
CT data set (20 images)	$256 \times 256 \times 8$	1.3	650	2 : 1

the display window and hence the number of pixels needed to output a frame. Naturally, the window size must be large enough to allow a valid teleconsultation to take place.

3.2.8   Telecommunications Standards

Clearly, for telemedicine to work, the units at both ends of the teleconferencing link must use the same codec algorithms and other transmission protocols. To ensure compatibility the United Nations *International Telecommunications Union* (ITU) has defined a range of standards to guarantee interoperability even if the videoconferencing equipment originates from different manufacturers. The most important standards are summarised in Table 3.3.

A useful summary of videoconferencing standards, including those for data and audio, is available in reference [109]. Reference [110] has an approachable account of the development of the H.xxx standards, showing the impact of packet switching on the Internet and the belated realisation that most videoconferencing takes place over the PSTN. Equipment that does not conform to the H.320 standard should be avoided.

Table 3.3.   Important ITU videoconferencing standards

Standard	Purpose
H.320	The oldest (1993) videoconferencing standards for communication over ISDN
H.323	An updated standard for videoconferencing over local area networks (LANs) and the Internet
H.324	A protocol for videoconferencing over the standard telephone network H.324 can also be used over ISDN so it may eventually supersede H.320
H.261	The codec defined in H.320 (for CIF images)
H.263	The codec defined in H.320 (for QCIF images)
T.120	A suite of protocols to allow concurrent users (multipoint data conferencing) to use whiteboards and annotation etc

3.3   TELECONSULATION SYSTEM COMPONENTS

3.3.1   The Building Blocks

There are many ways to distinguish the building blocks of a teleconsultation system. For simplicity, we shall employ a model that specifies the following four components:

- the videoconferencing system;
- multipoint systems;
- the image display system;
- telemonitoring devices.

The total cost of a teleconsultation site designed around these building blocks is typically US$ 50 000–100 000 [2]. Let us examine the components in more detail [21, 111].

3.3.2   The Videoconferencing System

This component is the (frequently commercially built) unit that organises the transmission, reception and storage of information from the teleconsultation process. Technology is advancing all of the time but currently we can identify four distinct types of system.

Rollabout Systems

These are self-contained, mobile units comprising a monitor or television screen atop a console containing the associated hardware. The console is fitted with wheels or castors, so that it can be moved between sites, and has sockets for local electrical connections.

Rollabout units, or group systems as they are sometimes known, produce high-quality sound and video and they are widely used in business.

Set-top Systems

As the name suggests, these units are also portable but miniaturisation puts all of the circuitry into a single box that sits on top of a conventional television set to give a system of moderate quality.

Desktop Systems

In these examples, the system box has been dispensed with and the circuitry has been located on a standard PC card for insertion into a desktop computer. In desktop videoconferencing (DVC), quality is sacrificed for convenience although utility is still high and cost is low.

Public Switched Telephone Network System

All of the above systems use digital telecommunications, often ISDN (see Section 3.4.3), but with better compression algorithms it has become possible to transmit video pictures across the public switched telephone network system. Picture quality is of course limited but connectivity is extremely high, allowing telemedicine to the home [112].

Irrespective of the type, a videoconferencing system consists of the same basic components:

- *Codec*, which, as we have seen, compresses and decompresses still and video images. The codec also manipulates the audio information and ensures synchronisation of voice and image. A further task is to control the interface between the videoconferencing unit and the network and peripherals.
- *Monitor*, to display video images either on a television or monitor according to the NTSC or PAL standards. Section 3.3.4 adds a little more to this description.
- *Camera*, usually an auto-focus, auto-iris, single chip device with remote pan/tilt/zoom to capture information from any part of the consultation room. The camera can be controlled locally or from the remote site.
- *Audio system*, which needs surprising sophistication to make it an acceptable approximation to normal speech. The system should provide automatic *echo correction* and allow *full duplex* conversation, i.e. the ability to interrupt and be interrupted. It should also have *automatic gain control* so that listeners can hear no matter how close or far a talker is from the microphone.
- *User interface* to make the system easy to operate for all users. A mouse or some other push-button control may be more acceptable than a keyboard.

The first commercial videoconferencing system was AT&T's Picturephone launched at the 1964 World Fair [113]. The telephone infrastructure at that time could not support the required transmission rates and sales were poor although the device was a clear 'proof of concept'. AT&T attempted to develop the idea in the late 1960s and early 1970s, including some telemedicine applications that showed what might be possible if the technology could be developed further.

The real breakthrough in mass-market terms was made in the early 1990s by Intel with its ProShare personal videoconferencing product designed to operate over ISDN networks. The market has since expanded to include PictureTel [114], VTEL and CLI, all of which offer a range of products and services to suit individual requirements.

3.3.3   Multipoint Systems

Most of our descriptions and examples of teleconsultation systems have assumed implicitly that there are two transmitting/receiving stations in the videoconferencing link-up. This is not a technological restriction, however, and multiple stations are quite possible.

The technical approach depends upon the telecommunications protocol. H.320 systems operating with the ISDN standard are essentially *point-to-point* systems and they need a hardware device known as a *multipoint control unit* to manage the ISDN lines and hold a multipoint conference. Alternatively, H.323 systems using Internet protocols require a hardware or software *multipoint conference server* to route the audio and video streams to the conference participants.

The approach and the videoconferencing standard adopted will often depend upon existing equipment but expert advice is necessary to avoid costly mistakes. Reference [115] has some useful comments on multipoint operation and the implication of the H.xxx standards for system choice. See also reference [116].

3.3.4   The Image Display System

The image display is a critical part of the teleconsultation system since it is the main substitute for the visual examination carried out by the physician in a face-to-face consultation. Technologists distinguish between *image fidelity* and *image information content*. Image fidelity describes the closeness to the original image, be it a view of a person's eye or an X-ray film. Fidelity can be described by physical measurements such as luminance, dynamic range, resolution and so on [104, 117].

Image information content is more subjective and reflects the amount of information needed to detect diagnostically important features [104]. The highest quality is often not necessary to acquire sufficient information for the desired purpose [117]. Since quality usually has a cost element to it, there is also financial benefit in choosing equipment that is 'fit for purpose'.

The ultimate determinants of video quality are image resolution and effective frame rate [111]. Display resolution is determined by both the digitising and display devices and the former is usually the higher of the two, making screen resolution the controlling factor.

As we have seen (Section 3.2.7), the effective frame rate, or *motion fidelity*, is determined by the frame rate transmitted by the codec and the bandwidth of the videoconferencing connection. Low bandwidth, giving rise to jerky motion, may be more disturbing in some circumstances than poor picture resolution, so a lower resolution can be tolerated provided the bandwidth is high enough. Under other conditions, e.g. the teledermatology example quoted earlier, the transmitted image is essentially still, and high resolution is paramount [118].

Remember also that the video camera [119] as well as the environment surrounding the display unit, e.g. the lighting and the acoustics [117], can also affect information retrieval.

3.3.5 Telemonitoring Devices

The main task in most teleconsultations is visual examination of a patient. Even in telepsychiatry, body language and disposition are important cues to the patient's mental condition. When, however, further diagnostic information is needed then it can be obtained from medical peripherals that act as telemonitoring devices.

Special versions of common instruments such as stethoscopes, blood pressure monitors [120] and microscopes have been designed so that their output in the form of audio, electrical or video signals can be fed directly into the videoconferencing system and retrieved at the remote site. Table 3.4 lists [111] some common instruments that can be used in this way.

Table 3.4. Medical instruments as telemonitoring devices (after Ash [111])

Type of device	Examples	
Common diagnostic devices	Stethoscope	Dermoscope
	Otoscope	Vital signs monitor
Common imaging devices	Echocardiogram	Ultrasound
	Angiogram	Microscope
Common surgical devices	Laparoscope	Duodenoscope
	Endoscope	Colonoscope

3.4 TELECOMMUNICATION OPTIONS

3.4.1 Service Considerations

In Section 3.3, we considered the equipment components needed at the transmitting/receiving stations in the videoconferencing link. Now it is time to look at how we connect the stations together, i.e. the network or telecommunications infrastructure. If the link is confined to a single site then it may be possible to install a local area network (LAN) system. More often than not, however, we need some form of wide area network (WAN) operating over extended distances.

Ultimately, the nature of the clinical information conveyed during the teleconsultation ordains the minimum bandwidth of the network. We have seen already the heavy demands that high definition images and video make on network bandwidth. If real-time requirements exceed the existing bandwidth then it may be necessary to revert to store-and-forward techniques or some other strategy to achieve the required utility. The alternative is to install a purpose-built infrastructure but this approach may be prohibitively expensive unless the cost can be shared with other users.

Bandwidth rates vary considerably from about 1.2 Kbps for some mobile telephones to 1000 Mbps for transmission through fibre-optic cables. Table 3.5 (after Falconer [21]) illustrates the range of options that we shall describe in this section, in order of increasing transfer rate.

The reliability of most of these different systems is extremely high especially now that much of the PSTN network is digital. The main operating problem arises with shared bandwidth systems such as the Internet, where the service can suffer if there is intensive traffic from other users. More modern protocols such as asynchronous transfer mode (ATM) can reserve bandwidth and release it on breaking the connection.

Let us look at some features of the options in Table 3.5, combining the last three entries under the heading of dedicated wide area connections. The Internet is dealt with throughout the book.

Table 3.5.   Telecommunication options (after Falconer [21])

System	Data transfer rate	Advantages/disadvantages
PSTN	56 Kbps	Cheap, ubiquitous
		Slow, not suitable for high resolution
ISDN (basic rate)	128 Kbps	Cheap, flexible
		Slow, patchy availability
ISDN (Primary rate)	< 2 Mbps	Fast, high quality
		Expensive, patchy availability
Satellite	< 2 Mbps	High quality, remote access
		Expensive
Wireless	< 2 Mbps	Convenience, free movement
		New technology, limited standards
Microwave	< 20 Mbps	Good quality, inexpensive to run
		Line of sight only, short distances
Leased lines	64 Kbps–50 Mbps	Reliable
		Expensive, inflexible
ATM, DSVD, ADSL	155 Mbps	High bandwidth
		Expensive, may be superseded

3.4.2   Public Switched Telephone Network

This low bandwidth option is still attractive because of its massive presence throughout the world. The theoretical bandwidth of 56 Kbps is only reached in the most well-maintained installations but in practice[2] is sufficient for audio, video and data sharing, especially when used with the latest high speed processors, compression algorithms and video display software.

If it were not for British Telecom's pricing structure, many UK users would have long since changed to ISDN, as they have done in other countries.

3.4.3 ISDN

Integrated services digital network (ISDN) is, as the name suggests, a purely digital service although it operates over standard telephone lines, effectively replacing the PSTN system. The *basic rate interface* (BRI) comprises two 64 Kbps (B) channels and a 16 Kbps data signal (D) channel. The *primary rate interface* (PRI) multiplies the number of B channels to up to 30 (in Europe) with a single 64 Kbps D channel.

Channels can be coupled together so that a two-channel BRI (ISDN-2) system can work at 128 Kbps and a six-channel PRI set-up can function at 384 Kbps, which is fast enough to provide smooth motion video under most circumstances [121]. Higher rate PRI lines can produce rates up to 2 Mbps, giving very high quality images.

ISDN connections are highly flexible since extra lines can be added later and the technology can be used for multipoint control (Section 3.3.3). It is often the first choice for telemedicine [21].

3.4.4 Satellite

Expense is the severest criticism of satellite systems but they can be used 'where no other technology can go'. This flexibility is truly global and the technology has been used to establish telemedical links in developing countries [9] as well as mobile links to areas where natural disasters have occurred [1].

Satellite connections are also the standard way to deal with emergencies onboard ships or in military theatres. As costs fall it seems likely that the technology will become increasing competitive and available for affordable, on-demand services [122, 123] as well as for mobile applications. Compression algorithms make a crucial contribution to these developments [123, 124].

---

[2] The quality of analogue telephone lines is rarely good enough to meet the V90 modem standard of 56 Kbps. The implementation is also an asymmetrical one, making use of digital land lines between exchanges and analogue lines from the exchange to the user. Thus, downstream transmission operates at 56 Kbps over the digital lines and at a lower speed over the analogue sections. The upstream section from the user to the exchange starts over analogue lines and cannot be accelerated. The consequence is a speed of roughly 45 Kbps for the downstream and 28.8 Kbps for the upstream lines.

Opportunities for healthcare distance learning broadcasts have also been realised [56].

3.4.5   Wireless Technologies

Wireless technologies have been a long time coming. Now they are developing rapidly, spurred on by the deluge of mobile telephones and the relentless advances that drive that market. Smaller and lighter devices, longer battery life, better user interfaces, lower costs and the establishment of communication standards have all contributed to the upsurge in sales and development.

In healthcare, where the workforce have always been mobile, the main drivers have been to help healthcare workers to communicate efficiently and to find ways to enter clinical and related data into computer systems at the point of origin. The electronic patient record, and access to it at any place and any time, especially during a consultation with a patient, is 'another force driving the acceptance of wireless technologies' [125].

Another sign of forthcoming maturity, the emergence of standards, took a leap forward in 1997 with the publication of the first *wireless Ethernet* standard, IEEE 802.11, although alternative technologies add some confusion for buyers [125]. One such technology, the Internet Protocol (IP), has led to a group of *voice-over-IP* products that integrate voice and data. Using this technology, one hospital has shut down its admissions department; patients are now assigned a room on entry and an admissions clerk visits them to take their details with a laptop computer equipped with a wireless LAN card [125].

Many observers see the future of wireless technologies as linked inextricably with the Internet. *Wireless application protocol* (WAP) [126, 127] is a set of protocols and global standards that bridge the gap between mobile devices such as telephones and the land-line infrastructure of the Internet. These standards include a wireless application environment (WAE) that opens the door for operators, manufacturers and content providers to develop value-added services without the need for additional infrastructure or equipment modifications.

Healthcare applications [128] include online information retrieval for physicians for test results or access to databases during ward rounds, two-way communication between carers and patients, for example, to alert patients to take prescribed medication and have them confirm their adherence, the reissue of prescriptions, and the communication of news about diseases or services.

In addition, the new *Bluetooth* technology [129] allows mobile devices to communicate with computers within a 10 m distance without physical connections, providing for patient monitoring and emergency alarms to remote locations.

These examples not only boost the efficiency of face-to-face medicine but they contribute to the new delivery paradigm of telemedicine, a development technically limited at present by low bandwidth communications links. The current *Global Service for Mobile Communications*[3] (GSM) technology does not permit mobile multimedia and web browsing but the advent of *General Packet Radio Service* (GPRS), and other technologies, will increase the bandwidth to 115 Kbps and above, rivalling fixed-line speeds [127, 130]. WAP may not translate desktop web browsing to the mobile telephone due to time and processing requirements but real-time voice and data transmission, and eventually real-time wireless video, will open many prospects for radical changes in telehealth delivery.

Over the horizon, a new breed of smart phones with HTML and personal digital assistant (PDA) capabilities is already threatening the WAP future before it becomes established [131].

3.4.6   Dedicated Wide Area Connections

The last three entries in Table 3.5 are all examples of dedicated wide area connections, i.e. those that are permanently devoted to organisational use rather than dial-on-demand use by the general public.

The first example, *microwave* connections, are expensive to install but cost very little to run. Bandwidth is high, typically 2–10 Mbps, but their chief disadvantage is that there must be an unobstructed line of sight between stations, meaning that the stations have to be less than 30 km apart, less in fog! Consequently, microwave networks are using LANs, often in urban areas, and connecting buildings on adjacent sites.

Leased lines are the oldest type of wide area connectivity and were installed by many large organisations during the 1980s. They are essentially private lines that offer direct, dedicated connections between points. The lines are leased monthly from a local or long-distance carrier and are priced on the basis of distance and bandwidth.

Bandwidths range from 64 Mbps (T0), through 1.55 Mbps (T1) to 45 Mbps (T3). A typical cost for a T3 line over a 350-mile distance is £20 000 per month with no extra charges for usage. Leased lines are attractive to organisations with stringent security requirements and very high usage rates, where dial-on-demand would be more expensive.

Asynchronous transfer mode (ATM) is a cell relay technology [132] that uses fixed-length data packets and transmits these asynchronously by dropping them into available cells as they pass (as on a fixed-speed conveyor belt) the transmitting station. The speed of transmission adapts to the available bandwidth of the media (twisted pair, coaxial, optical) so that ATM buffers data

---

[3] The original meaning of GSM is Group Spécial Mobile, which is the name of a study group set up in 1982 by the Conference of European Posts and Telegraphs (CEPT) to develop a pan-European public land mobile communications system.

and can send voice, data and video over mid-speed (56 Kbps to 1.5 Mbps) lines or high speed (155 Mbps) lines and even at multi-gigabit per second rates.

Because of its flexibility and speed, ATM could become the single, all-embracing technology for corporate communications. Its progress to date has been hampered by cost and the lack of voice and video transmission standards so that most implementations are proprietary, i.e. the equipment at either end of the line has to be purchased from the same supplier and the line may not connect with lines supported by other ATM suppliers.

There have been very few telemedicine applications with ATM and it may be hijacked before it makes its presence felt by newer technologies such as *digital simultaneous voice and data* (DSVD) and *asymmetric digital subscriber line* (ADSL). These are data/voice line-sharing techniques [133] like ISDN. Like ATM, they operate over unshielded twisted pair lines and in this respect are less demanding than ISDN, which often needs newer, higher quality lines to make it work satisfactorily.

DSVD is a modem technology that runs voice and data over a single telephone line. Users at both ends of the line must have a DSVD modem. DSVD was developed to improve services to home and mobile users. ADSL has a different purpose, to provide high bandwidth for video-on-demand services. Such services are inherently unidirectional and the transmission return rate is much slower than the forward one—hence the term 'asymmetric' in the title. A typical ADSL configuration operating over unshielded twisted pair offers a forward stream rate of 6 Mbps (9 Mbps is the theoretical limit) and a return rate of 64 Kbps. At this rate the forward stream can support four channels of compressed video while simultaneously using the return channel for communication.

Telecommunications technologies have a habit of leap-frogging one another and new examples seem to multiply existing transmission rates by orders of magnitude. It's an exciting time for telemedicine but it's difficult to keep up!

One thing missing from this book so far is a diagram so here is one to redress the omission. Figure 3.1 shows an example [134] of how the various telecommunications technologies can be integrated into a healthcare network based on telemedicine principles. Connectivity is according to appropriateness and need so that service requirements are met while costs are controlled.

Figure 3.1 raises issues concerning the integration and operation of tele-medicine so we will finish the chapter by looking at some of the technological aspects of these issues. The issues we discuss are:

- systems integration;
- store-and-forward operation;
- real-time operation.

Chapter 5 will deal with the organisational aspects of introducing and oper-ating telemedicine services.

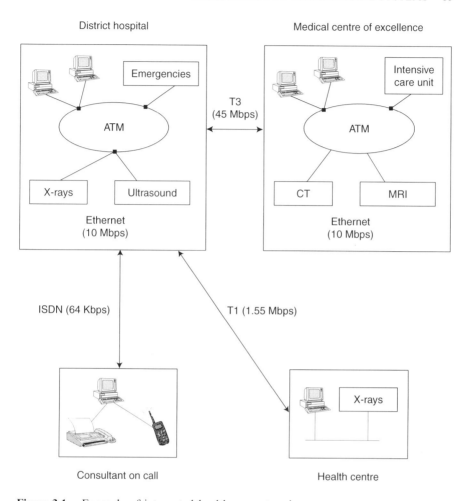

Figure 3.1. Example of integrated healthcare network

3.5 INTEGRATION AND OPERATIONAL ISSUES

3.5.1 Systems Integration

Most developed societies distinguish three sectors for the delivery of health-care to their citizens. Although titles and practices differ, the first contact patients usually have with healthcare professionals is with general practitioners in the primary sector, who refer them if necessary to hospital consultants in the secondary sector. Upon discharge from hospital, the recovering patient may need further therapy and support in the community or tertiary sector.

Although this model is simplistic it instantly reveals the distributed, and often hierarchical, nature of healthcare and the importance of information transmission and sharing. GPs need to communicate with hospitals, hospitals are set up to serve local, regional and national needs as well as to concentrate on certain specialities, and community health organisations must deal with patients in their own homes. Even within the hospital, the most compact and integrated environment for patient care, there are many different systems that need to operate together to deliver an efficient health service.

Systems integration is therefore a crucial issue for clinicians, managers and information system technologists, as well as for patients. Uncoordinated planning and legacy and proprietary systems with limited or no networking capabilities present major challenges to systems integration. It is essential, however, that the process of upgrading these systems and services plans for the future provision of telemedical facilities.

What telemedical issues need to be considered in this planning process? Only recently have healthcare professionals begun to address this question [89–91]. Here are some suggestions from the systems integration perspective.

Plan for Future Needs Not Present Ones

This may seem an obvious statement but the implications of not doing it make its repetition worth while. Future needs may include upgraded or new services that have more demanding bandwidth requirements than present ones, and the wrong decision may necessitate ripping out the old network to install a new one. Irrespective of clinical services, computer technology changes so rapidly that it is almost inevitable that equipment will need replacement on a regular basis.

Because of this, and similar advances in medical technology and treatment, it is very difficult to predict accurately future needs and demands. The sensible telemedicine strategist will therefore build flexible, standardised systems that can be upgraded incrementally with minimum disruption. Purchasing systems for current needs but ensuring that they can be updated for future ones also spreads costs and harnesses, rather than falls victim to, the march of technology.

Adopt Open Systems Technologies

Open systems [135] technologies have been around for nearly 15 years now but there are still IT directors and managers who have yet to subscribe to their benefits. The concept of open systems is based on the premise that a piece of computer equipment from one manufacturer should work with a piece of equipment from another company, i.e. there should be no need to buy equipment from a sole supplier. System standards, whether *de jure* (e.g. Ethernet) or *de facto* (e.g. Microsoft Windows), have done a lot to promote this concept but manufacturers, e.g. of videoconferencing equipment, do have a tendency to tweak interfaces or other features to 'improve performance'.

The three characteristics of open systems [135] are:

- *interoperability*: the ability of hardware and software to work together;
- *portability*: the ability of software designed for one computer platform to work on others;
- *scalability*: the ability of software to function properly on both small and large systems.

These characteristics should be uppermost in the mind of telemedicine strategists as they plan new systems and services.

Plan Links with the Electronic Patient Record

While enthusiasts sing the praises of telemedicine, the real benefits will only become evident when the healthcare professional has the patient's full and current medical record available before or at the time of the teleconsultation [37]. This is only possible if the patient history is maintained electronically so that the record can be referred to during the consultation and updated during the teleconsultation or after it ends. Software can be written to automate these processes and ease the administrative burden.

To be effective, the information held on the electronic patient record (EPR) must be comprehensive and easily accessible. It must also be available when needed in case of emergency and this requirement implies a suitable network infrastructure and protocols allowing transmission of the data to the point of need, wherever the data are held. Ideally, the EPR also has links to scientific knowledge databases, e.g. to support clinical decision making and the pre-scription of generic and cost-effective drugs.

These requirements, and the difficulty of achieving them, raise the EPR to holy grail status. However, progress is being made [37, 136, 137], particularly in the USA where the billing requirement ensures that itemised treatments and outcomes are recorded on the American equivalent, the computerised medical record (CMR). Interestingly, reimbursement of costs is only fully allowable for face-to-face, rather then telemedicine, consultations but this situation will change.

3.5.2 Store-and-Forward Operation

Store-and-forward operation refers to situations in which information has been prerecorded [108] before transmission and reception, i.e. the information is not transferred during the teleconsultation. Such processes are anything but new, as the general postal service and the modern equivalent, courier services, demonstrate.

Diagnosis and clinical monitoring are the main applications of store-and-forward operation. The approach is used when all of the information needed for a satisfactory teleconsultation can be acquired without any intervention on the part of the person receiving it [108]. The value of the EPR in this circumstance is immediately obvious. Email is currently a useful alternative.

An advantage of store-and-forward operation is that the link between sites does not need to be operational at all times. Instead, the information is transmitted to a store-and-forward server (perhaps a mail server) and the recipient accesses the server and downloads the information at his or her later convenience. An added benefit of this approach is the ability to combine information from several sources and receive it at a single time. Alternatively, a single piece of information can be sent to the server and accessed from several sites at convenient times.

In Section 3.2, we identified the various types of information used in telemedicine and distinguished text and data, audio, still images and video. Store-and-forward mode is used mostly for text and data and still image transmissions. Text and data are frequently sent by modem or fax, or increasingly via the Internet. Digitised electrocardiographs (ECGs) [138] and electroencephalograms (EEGs) [139] are the most common examples in this category.

Teleradiology [104] is by far the most practised instance of store-and-forward operation with still images. Other 'teles' include telepathology [140], teledermatology [119] and tele-ophthalmology [141]. Good results have been obtained with radiology and dermatology studies but technology and practice have still some way to go before telepathology is as successful [142].

3.5.3   Real-time Telemedicine

Real-time telemedicine occurs when the transmitted information is received in the same teleconsultation session [143]. Real-time teleconsultation allows interaction between the transmitter and the recipient of the information and is used when an immediate outcome is needed, e.g. in an emergency. Delays are avoided and the real-time interaction between the patient/healthcare professional and the consultant also provides an educational benefit. The cost of these benefits is reflected in the need for higher bandwidth than is required for store-and-forward operation.

Real-time telemedicine makes use of all of the data types that we have identified. Audio data are most commonly transmitted in telephone conversations for a whole raft of purposes ranging from diagnosis, through monitoring, to patient support. Examples of data and text transfer have been given already in our discussion [111] on telemonitoring (Section 3.3.5). Mobile telephones with graphical displays can now be used to transmit ECGs [144].

Still image transfer in real time is also apparent in the disciplines noted for store-and-forward operation [145, 146], including a long-standing telepathology service in Norway [146], and mobile telephones are again having an impact [147]. However, it is with video transfer that real-time telemedicine comes into is own. Telepsychiatry [148] is one of the earliest and probably the most successful applications [149] since it is difficult to do in store-and-forward mode. Similarly, accident and emergency telemedicine [150] must be done in real-time since delays are unacceptable.

3.6   SUMMARY

In Chapter 3 we have seen that:

- Telemedicine information is of four distinct types; text and data, audio, still (single) images and video (sequential) images.
- Bandwidth is the capacity of a transmission medium to carry information.
- Video images conform to the National Television Standards Committee (NTSC) or Phase Alternating Line (PAL) standards. The Common Intermediate Format (CIF) is a format introduced to provide compatibility between NTSC and PAL.
- Still images and video file sizes can be large, and transmission times and costs are reduced by data compression. Image compression may be lossless, without loss of data on decompression, or lossy, in which event data are lost on compression and cannot be recovered by decompression.
- Lossless and lossy compression achieve compression ratios of up to 3 : 1 and 100 : 1, respectively.
- Video frame rates of 25 discrete pictures per second give the illusion of continuous motion. At lower rates, the sequence of events on screen can appear discontinuous and jerky, an effect known as motion artefact.
- Important videoconferencing standards are H.320, the oldest videoconferencing standard for communication over ISDN, H.323, an updated standard for videoconferencing over local area networks (LANs) and the Internet, and H.324, a protocol for videoconferencing over the standard telephone network.
- The components of a telemedicine system include the videoconferencing system, multi-point systems, the image display system and telemonitoring devices.
- Telecommunication options for telemedicine include, in order of increasing bandwidth, the public switched telephone network (PSTN), ISDN, satellite, wireless technologies, microwave, leased lines, ATM, DSVD and ADSL.
- Systems integration issues are important when planning a telemedicine service.
- Store-and-forward systems are used for diagnosis and clinical monitoring when all of the information needed for a satisfactory teleconsultation can be acquired without any intervention on the part of the person receiving it.
- The main advantage of store-and-forward operation is that the link between sites does not need to be operational at all times. Instead, the

information is transmitted to a store-and-forward server and the recipient accesses the server at his or her later convenience.

- Real-time telemedicine occurs when the transmitted information is received in the same teleconsultation session. It is used when an immediate outcome is needed, e.g. in an emergency. The approach needs higher bandwidth than store-and-forward operation.
- Real-time telemedicine is most necessary for the transmission of video images.

4

TELEMEDICINE SERVICE PROVIDERS AND APPLICATIONS

OBJECTIVES

At the end of this chapter you should be able to:

- describe the main telemedicine services in the primary sector;
- describe the main telemedicine services in the secondary sector;
- describe the telecare services in the community sector;
- describe the uses of telemedicine by ambulance organisations;
- describe the uses of telemedicine by pharmacists;
- describe the uses of telemedicine by managed care organisations;
- describe the uses of telemedicine by transport operators;
- describe the uses of telemedicine by the military and space agencies;
- describe the uses of telemedicine by non-governmental organisations.

4.1   INTRODUCTION

Chapter 4 describes the main users and applications of telemedicine. Several of the practitioners and their applications have been mentioned in earlier chapters. Hence, Chapter 4 also gives us an opportunity to tidy up some loose ends before we look at the design and implementation of telemedicine services in Chapter 5.

The layout of the present chapter is very simple. We divide users into two groups. The first comprises what we might call mainstream healthcare services. It deals with GPs and hospital clinicians and also describes community sector professionals who provide telecare services. Ambulance services and pharmacists are also included.

The second group looks mainly at commercial companies, and governmental and not-for-profit agencies. Examples cover managed care organisations, transport operators, and military and space agencies. There is considerable overlap both between and within groups arising from the strong interaction between carers and the delivery of integrated care.

The discussion tries to draw out some general principles and experience from telemedicine and telecare practice as well as illustrating users and applications.

4.2   MAINSTREAM HEALTH SECTOR SERVICES

4.2.1   General Practitioners and Primary Care Services

The potential for telemedicine in primary care is yet to be realised [73]. Much of the GP's work is concerned with minor ailments and it seems likely that the majority of these will continue to be diagnosed by patients presenting themselves at the surgery or health centre. Increasingly, however, we shall see surgeries cropping up in public areas such as shopping malls. Does the physician need to be on the premises? Dr Woodrow Kessler from Media, Pennsylvania thinks not [85].

Dr Kessler has a walk-in surgery in a mall in Philadelphia. Patients enter the surgery and register with a nurse, who asks a series of diagnostic questions prompted by a computer. The nurse reads the positive answers to Dr Kessler or one of his partners at the other end of a videoconferencing link and, with the nurse's help, the doctor examines the patient with simple tools such as a laryngoscope or otoscope. He then states his diagnosis and care plan. Cost? $15 for five minutes! No insurance, cash on the nail!

This is convenience medicine. Patients do not have to make a special appointment, take time off work, or take a detour to the surgery. They can pop in during their lunch break or after work. For the minor complaints it is meant to deal with it is ideal. In addition, it takes pressure off the mainstream health services and helps them to deal effectively with more serious conditions.

We have not seen this approach in the UK yet but it is coming [151].

In a more conventional vein we can distinguish three main ways in which GPs can use clinical telemedicine to benefit patients and themselves:

- monitoring of conditions;
- minor injuries and emergencies;
- better coordination with secondary care.

Monitoring of Conditions

Once the GP has established the diagnosis and the care plan, it is often necessary to monitor the treatment to see how the patient is responding. This requirement often means an inconvenient or even difficult trip to the surgery to check blood pressure or some other straightforward measurement. Better if the measurement can be made at home and transmitted to the doctor via telephone, fax or email.

This is the telemonitoring scenario we described in Section 2.2.3, hypertension [65] and diabetes mellitus [66] being the most common conditions to be treated in this way. A video link is not necessary for this type of routine monitoring but there is some concern about the accuracy of patient-administered tests, which could be reduced if healthcare workers could observe the patients as they performed the test and advise them on technique [152].

Minor Injuries and Emergencies

Once again the stress here is on the word 'minor'. Reference [153] describes an often-quoted study on telemedical support of a minor treatment centre (MTC) in London. MTCs were a government initiative intended as walk-in centres for the 20–40% of patients who unnecessarily attended traditional Accident and Emergency (A&E) departments. The South Westminster Centre for Health MTC was set up following closure of the local hospital and movement of its A&E department elsewhere.

A video link using basic-rate ISDN (Section 3.4.3) was established with the A&E department at Victoria Hospital, Belfast. In the first 12 months of the link, the MTC saw 9972 patients; 1.5% were referred to the local A&E department and 3.8% to their own GP. Only 0.5% were assessed using the telemedicine link. This relatively small number was attributed in part to the skilling of the MTC nurses, who learned so much from the early teleconsultations that they no longer needed to refer patients to doctors at the Victoria Hospital. A careful analysis of costs showed that the link produced a saving of about £42 000 per annum.

The skilling effect noted in this study is an interesting example of tele-education removing the need for the link. This educational aspect is one of the main reasons for GP interest in telemedicine.

Reference [154] describes a clinical evaluation of a minor injuries emergency department in an acute hospital using both real-time and store-and-forward videoconferencing. Teleconsultation was felt to assist decision making for remote practitioners, particularly for the real-time treatment of minor injuries.

Better Coordination with Secondary Care

Integrated care as advocated in the UK government White Paper *The New NHS* [36] can be facilitated by video links between primary care workers, hospital specialists and patients, allowing them to meet in a virtual clinic [155]. The clinic can take place in the GP's surgery, reducing waiting times and inconvenience to all parties. The tele-education component is also a bonus.

The cost of installing such a link would only be justified if the link were used for other purposes. Planning a portfolio of telemedical services is an important prerequisite in establishing the business case for expenditure and installation in GP surgeries (see Section 5.4).

An interesting study by Harno *et al.* [156] continues the Scandinavian concern with careful evaluation and cost effectiveness in telemedicine. The 18-month study investigated the use of telemedicine in medical outpatient clinics in two acute hospitals linked to three primary care centres. A total of 292 patients were referred and the authors' analysis showed that teleconsultations decreased both the number of essential referrals and the cost of treatment when referral was judged necessary.

Hjelm [73] gives other examples of the use of telemedicine in primary care.

4.2.2 Acute Hospital and Secondary Care Services

Throughout the book we have given numerous examples of the many applications of telemedicine in the acute hospital environment and there is no need to repeat our review here. Instead, Table 4.1 summarises our discussion and adds a few more examples with suitable and recent references.

We can, however, extract some general principles from these and other studies. First, the establishment of hospital–patient links where patients are able to spend more time in their own homes (telecare) is a major benefit in many cases. This is no more obvious than in the extensive teledialysis work centred on The Queen Elizabeth Hospital (TQEH) in Adelaide, South Australia [48, 160]. Patients who would find it difficult to travel to Adelaide can carry out their own dialysis at home and communicate with clinicians and nurses at TQEH via a videoconferencing link. This interaction builds confidence, self-reliance and independence.

Second, inter-hospital links offer improved cover and specialist advice. For example, the teaching hospital in Lund in Sweden provides an out-of-hours teleradiology service to 11 local hospitals [161]. Third, acute hospitals can provide valuable support for practitioners in remote areas such as the Antarctic [162].

Fourth, while visual contact always enhances communication (as in the renal dialysis example) there are certain disciplines where it is essential in order to pick up facial expressions and body language. Psychiatry is one such area. McLaren [163] has used simulated interviews in telepsychiatry to develop a better understanding of interpersonal communication, both face to face and mediated, and has suggested that the results could be used to train carers and maximise the therapeutic benefits of telemedicine.

We should add to this list the continuing staff development and medical and patient [164] education that attends almost all telemedicine projects and is the major role of teaching hospitals. The last point is obviously a consequence of funding models as well as of research activity and specialist expertise.

Table 4.1.   Specialist telemedicine services in the acute hospital environment

Teledermatology [47]	Telecardiology [144]
Telenephrology [48]	Telepsychiatry [148]
Teleradiology [104]	Accident and Emergency [150]
Teleneurophysiology [139]	Tele-obstetrics [157]
Tele-ophthalmology [141]	Tele-oncology [158]
Telepathology [142]	Tele-ENT [159]

4.2.3   Community Sector and Telecare Services

Many of the telemedicine outreach services we have mentioned from primary and secondary care to patients in their homes can be regarded as telecare services. Others could easily be extended in this way. In this section we shall take these examples as read and concentrate instead on services involving community carers.

In addition to the medical and technological drivers of healthcare, telecare often has a social aspect to it as housing authorities and social service departments seek to discharge their duty of care to residents in the community. Not surprisingly, elderly people are major users of telecare and the European Union has funded extensive programmes under the TIDE (telematics in support of the disabled and elderly) initiative [165, 166].

The clearest example of the relationship between the medical and social elements of care is the domiciliary visit by community nurses or midwives to patients confined to their homes. Although effective, this is an expensive way of delivering healthcare and prone to cutbacks. These cutbacks create a tension within a health service that wants to develop care-in-the-community, and among patients who increasingly see hospitalisation as an unattractive option.

There are many ongoing projects to improve the efficiency of domiciliary visits. For example, in Melbourne, Australia, the Royal District Nursing Service has equipped all of its nurses with laptop computers linked to mobile telephones so that data required for the visit are to hand and information obtained during the visit can be entered and transmitted to base quickly and easily [167]. As a result, all authorised carers have access to up-to-date information on all patients. With increased efficiency the nurse can either spend more time with a patient or see more patients in a day, or both.

Home healthcare is one of the most rapidly growing segments of the US healthcare market [168]. A pilot study [169] in Minneapolis used a purpose-designed Personal Telemedicine Unit (PTU) operating over the widely available analogue telephone network. Patients had no difficulty with the technology or with televisiting. The average charge for a televisit was $15 as opposed to $90 for a physical visit including travelling costs. In one instance, telecare allowed a patient to stay in her own home for six months whereas a nursing home stay would have cost $18 000. The cost of the six-month telecare service was $2000. Other cases show improved medicines compliance and a reduction in hospitalisation.

Another alternative to the domiciliary visit is the 'smart house' [170, 171] where a range of simple sensors (e.g. door opening, toilet use, cooker use etc.) is fitted to monitor patient activity. A study by the University of New South Wales [172] in which four patients were monitored for five months revealed that some patients had undiagnosed medical problems that could be detected by home monitoring.

A final example demonstrates the diversity of telecare services. Italy has a hospital-at-home service which focuses on palliative care. A recent project [173] has looked at the use of video communications to improve the care of advanced cancer patients, prevent or avoid hospital admission, and improve communication between healthcare professionals and between patients, informal carers and healthcare professionals. Reference [174] describes a home-based tele-hospice service.

So what can we learn from these studies? A substantial point is that telecare can be used as a substitute for a significant fraction of home nursing visits [175]. An important outcome is that by caring for patients in their own homes we are frequently satisfying their wish to be in familiar surroundings with easy access to friends and relatives. Telecare therefore contributes to the quality and dignity of their lives. At the same time, it reduces healthcare costs and the burden on hospital beds and services as well as the quality of clinical outcomes [176].

Another interesting and supportive outcome is the finding that patients, even the elderly, seem to have little difficulty with the technology. Indeed, where the facility is available they often use it not only for direct communication with their formal carers but with the informal circle of carers who visit, run errands and help in other ways. It is obviously good to view as well as to chat!

Finally, the observation that telecare helps patients keep to their drug regimes is important since non-compliance is a common cause of delayed recovery or relapse, as well as being a waste of resources.

4.2.4 Ambulance Services

In an emergency, ambulance organisations and paramedics are invariably the first points of contact that patients have with formal treatment to improve their condition. Ambulance teams are therefore crucial to the recovery process since the first few minutes after the emergency occurs are often the critical period needed to stabilise patients and prepare them for further treatment.

Where time is of the essence, the chances of full recovery are greatly enhanced if the paramedic team can contact the emergency room so that doctors can assess the patient's condition, make the relevant decisions and have the appropriate staff and equipment ready on arrival. Equally important is the advice that doctors can give to the paramedic team if the emergency requires intervention beyond the team's normal expertise. Clearly, tele-medicine has a role to play here.

The impact of telemedicine actually begins before the ambulance is despatched. Telephone triage dealing with emergency calls for ambulances is now standard practice in the UK [177] as elsewhere to reduce the number of unnecessary calls, which can be as high as 50%.

However, real clinical benefits arise when telemedicine is used to reduce the time that the emergency room team needs to assess the patient. A video camera in the ambulance can allow hospital physicians to see a patient's physical condition while audio communication can relay information about heart rate, blood pressure and even blood analysis. Stroke and heart attack victims are some of the main beneficiaries of this new approach [178], which is applicable whether the ambulance is land-based or airborne. The military applications are obvious (see also Section 4.3.3).

4.2.5 Pharmacy Services

The link between telemedicine and pharmaceutical dispensing may not seem too obvious but we have come a long way since the telephone poison control centres of the 1950s [179]. Telepharmacy is now big business. In the USA, so-called Internet pharmacies allow patients to buy prescribed drugs online at discount prices. When, the healthcare system requires the patient to pay the full price of medication it pays to shop around to find the best price.

While the law is quite clear that only medication that has been properly prescribed by a certified physician can be purchased in this way, there are apparently increasing numbers of fly-by-night companies [180] that are prepared to sell anything to anyone. The legal companies want tighter regulation.

Pharmacists are only just beginning to consider the impact of telemedicine. Since patients do not need to see the doctor for a repeat prescription, they are now asking why they need to see the pharmacist to get the drugs. Alterna-tively, if you are in the drug store or chemist's shop, why not contact your doctor over the Internet, prove your identity, get your repeat prescription printed out and pick up the drugs on the spot.

Clearly, there are many issues of ethics, security and confidentiality, reimbursement and funding to be sorted out but the convenience factor will drive solutions in the e-health direction. A voluminous article [181] with the title 'Telemedicine and telepharmacy: current status and future implications' says more about the former than the latter but it is a good source of material.

That concludes our survey of telemedicine in the mainstream health sector. To end our discussion we turn our attention to the services offered by the commercial sector and other agencies.

4.3   COMMERCIAL SERVICES AND OTHER AGENCIES

4.3.1   Managed Care Organisations

The idea behind managed care is simple: those who pay the medical bills want to be sure that money is spent as efficiently as possible. In a fee-for-service system this is difficult to achieve because care is determined by physicians whose pay depends on how much treatment they provide. Managed care [182] has its origins in the insurance sector where the insurance companies pay the medical bills. In the USA, where managed care began, these companies began to hire doctors and nurses to offer second opinions and challenge the physicians' bills. To counteract these challenges, doctors and hospitals began to form group practices that provided planned and cost-conscious care.

The insurance cover offered by these managed care organisations therefore assumes a more active role in 'managing' their members' health than traditional insurance companies, which simply acted as intermediaries in the financial transactions. Gradually, some of the group practices evolved into health maintenance organisations (HMOs) [183] that cover all necessary medical services for a fixed pre-paid fee. HMOs are therefore organisations that both finance and deliver healthcare.

Whatever its precise form, a managed care organisation (MCO) has as its main objective the delivery of high-quality and cost-effective healthcare. Telemedicine and telecare seem to offer the prospect of achieving this delicate balance [34, 184]. Quality is enhanced by the availability of expert opinion, teleconferencing between clinicians, electronic information exchange, and continuing medical education. Cost effectiveness is realised by speedy billing and other electronic transactions.

The major driver for both quality enhancement and cost savings, however, is the reduction of use and stay in hospital, and recuperation in the patient's home. This is where telecare comes into its own with the ability to monitor a patient's progress and recall the patient to hospital only if the symptoms demand it.

Kansas seems to be a hot-bed of initiatives in the managed care/telemedicine arena. MCO, Saint Luke's Shawnee Mission Health System, has teamed up with a leading telecommunications provider, Sprint, to launch a telemedicine programme involving its seven hospitals [185]. The first video-conferencing phase was used for medical education and rounds. Subsequent phases have introduced teleradiology and the transmission of ultrasounds and electrocardiograms, and equipped nurses with portable monitoring units fitted with a camera so that clinical data transmissions and remote consults can occur between patients and their physicians.

Kansas Blue Cross, with 700 000 enrolled members throughout the state, has undertaken a project to cut expenses and improve care to chronically ill patients [186]. The MCO has developed a PSTN-based telemedicine system to reach out to homebound patients living in small towns and isolated areas. The aim is to reduce outpatient costs and provide more home visits for the same budget. A key factor in the scheme is the decision to reimburse clients for telemedicine-mediated home visits, and the company hopes to create a model for other MCOs.

Another feature of managed care plans looks set to create interest in telemedicine and telecare. The plans emphasise preventive treatment on the grounds that it is better to keep people healthy rather than wait to treat them when they get sick. The extension of this thesis has led to the concept of disease management [187].

Disease management is based on the premise that systematic, integrated, and evidence-based, long-term care of populations of patients with chronic, high-cost diseases (e.g. asthma, back pain, rheumatoid arthritis, dementia and diabetes) is more effective than episodic fragmented care of individuals. The incidence of acute episodes and complications associated with disease is reduced and quality of life improves. Better health outcomes reduce costs. Setting up 'disease management' programmes that operate across the boundaries of primary, secondary and community care requires high capital investment and state-of-the-art information technology. Few healthcare providers can readily supply these. Pharmaceutical industries can; hence the logic of contracting out services or setting up joint ventures [188].

In the UK, this is a paradigm shift in thinking about how a national health service should be financed. Given the perpetual crisis in the NHS, however, it seems almost inevitable, and certainly the holistic concept of disease management seems to make a lot of sense. Identification of the roles of telemedicine and telecare in disease management is at an early stage [189]. However, the expert opinion and exchange of information facilitated by telemedicine plus the integrated care into the community favoured by telecare would appear to offer many opportunities.

MCOs have been quick to grasp that the benefits of telemedicine and telecare will only be fully realised if these approaches are linked to the development of the electronic medical record. An interesting PhD thesis by Dalton [190] explores this relationship and suggests that multidisciplinary working is central to success, as is the management of change.

4.3.2 Transport Services

We have already mentioned (Section 1.4.2) healthcare for travellers as a driver of interest in telemedicine. The concern, as with rural or disadvantaged populations, is to improve the quality of healthcare or make it available where none existed previously. The scenario is usually one of a clear emergency or of the need for advice and back-up to deal with conditions that could range from trivial to serious.

We can perceive two main thrusts in what we can refer to as mobile telemedicine. The first is a strategic one; that is, to develop an organisational approach to dealing with events that can swing into action when the events occur. This requirement suggests the establishment of some sort of infra-structure and guidelines or protocols for handling diagnosis and treatment. The second thrust is the development of telemonitoring devices to extend the range of vital signs that can be transmitted to specialist centres to improve diagnosis and delivery of the care plan.

Let us look at two examples that illuminate these concepts.

The first is illustrated by the EU-funded NIVEMES (Network of Integrated Vertical Medical Services) Project established in 1996 for a period of three years. NIVEMES [191] sets out to develop an international telemedicine network of healthcare service providers aimed at the provision of high-quality diagnosis or first-level assistance. The first phase concentrated on the shipping sector and on remote populations of small islands as well as on disaster regions without normal telecommunications services.

The project network consists of a coherent assembly of 15 healthcare and telecommunications providers and transport experts from five EU countries. Ships' officers receive training to use an on-board computer and transmission system that can transfer patients' medical data to mainland healthcare organ-isations via satellite links.

The telemedicine services are divided into scheduled or emergency accord-ing to the facilities at the local medical centre. They include:

- regular check-ups covering activities otherwise provided by mobile services;
- planned check-ups of remote populations;
- diagnostic evaluations based on available data;
- emergency services, including urgent evaluations and transfer decisions.

The origins of NIVEMES go back a long way (Section 1.3.1) and there is much experience on which to build success.

The second example illustrates the technological advances in telemonitoring that have been applied to air travel. Like its competitors, British Airways is concerned to provide the best available healthcare to its passengers [192]. Each aircraft carries a comprehensive medical kit and trained personnel but the situation in a Boeing 747 at 30 000 feet on a 17-hour long-haul flight is not exactly equivalent to a fully-equipped emergency room on the ground.

Since the 1980s, commercial companies based in hospitals have operated a verbal support service for in-flight emergencies. However, question-and-answer techniques are no substitute for measurements and so BA has worked with Telemedic Systems to develop a laptop computer device to monitor vital signs and relay them to medical personnel on the ground via satellite [193]. Telemedic Systems has worked with similar companies to add new monitors to the basic vital signs unit.

For example, patients now have access to a respiratory device that measures air mass flow and analyses their breath since the latter can reveal the incidence of such conditions as diabetes, liver disease or an acute myocardial infarction. A second device monitors pupil dilation, which is an indicator for several conditions, including the seriousness of head injuries.

Naturally, diagnosis is more secure if the physician can see the patient, and this is now possible via the transmission of highly compressed video signals [112] using cellular networks and satellite hook-ups. The time may not be too far away when airlines offer a range of emergency services tailored to the class of ticket you buy—a heart transplant in first class and an aspirin in economy!

4.3.3   Space and Military Agencies

In many respects, space and military applications of telemedicine are leading edge in the sense that they are practised in the most demanding and adverse circumstances. They are unusual in other respects too.

Both astronauts and military personnel are by their profession extremely fit, and the incidence of certain types of illness, e.g. chronic conditions, is low. In astro-telemedicine, if an astronaut does fall sick then it may be some time before he or she can return to earth for treatment. In-flight and hence (very) remote treatment is therefore highly reliable although the conditions are likely to be very different to those found on the planet surface. In terrestrial war zones, an injured combatant can be evacuated for further treatment but the priority may be to return him or her to active duty as soon as possible.

Clearly, astro- and military telemedicine demand rapid diagnosis and treatment in far from ideal circumstances. The use of telemedicine is a necessity, not an option. Interestingly, however, the different needs of space and military medicine have made telemedicine develop from different starting points.

In astro-telemedicine, the assumption is that the astronaut will not be subject to physical injury (although this assumption is begin revised as the space walk become more common and space stations become more than a part of science fiction). Instead, ground control is more concerned about how individuals react to space conditions and how to deal with illness and disease should they occur.

The US National Aeronautics and Space Administration (NASA), which has led the expansion of space travel, has therefore pioneered research and development into biosensors [194] and the associated telemetry. With the experience gained, NASA is now turning its attention to the miniaturisation of devices and their integration into health management systems. These systems display patient information, including video and audio, and provide access to computerised patient records, electronic medical books and literature, and decision support systems—a veritable hospital in a box. The outcomes are already filtering into everyday, terrestrial medicine.

Military action is no less dangerous than space flight but potentially much more violent. The treatment of physical injury and trauma has therefore been the guiding principle in the development of military telemedicine. Although the circumstances in a mobile army surgical hospital (MASH) are a lot less luxurious than an insurance-funded bed in a private hospital, it is also common practice to have surgeons and some specialists on site to deal with cases.

Military telemedicine has another advantage (if that is the right word) over its astro-cousin, in that its patient base is much bigger. This fact allows it to use telemedicine in a more predictive way. For example, during and after the Gulf War, large numbers of soldiers developed symptoms that failed to yield to conventional medicine, the so-called 'Gulf syndrome' classified by the military as a 'disease non-battle injury'.

The US Air Force chiefs, concerned about the environment they had to draft personnel into, developed Desert Care [195], a data warehouse system populated with anonymised records for previously and currently active personnel, and information on the terrain and local conditions. Now, when a serviceman or woman consults a doctor, this system can be queried to see if other personnel have presented similar symptoms and if there is any underlying pattern such as exposure to some environmental hazard. In effect, Desert Care becomes an online tool for revealing trends and allowing commanders to take the necessary action.

The UK military services have not had the funding to embark upon such cutting-edge developments. However, telemedicine has been used successfully in Bosnia [196] and other conflict areas, and efforts have been made to include it in the Surgeon General's Information Strategy.

Because of their access to facilities, particularly satellite technology [197], and experience in emergencies, space and military agencies are often the first to be called in when there is some sort of natural catastrophe such as an earthquake or flood. Again with lessons learned, agencies are now planning appropriate responses in advance of disasters and developing telemedicine solutions at all stages [198, 199].

4.3.4 Community Alarm Services

This may seem a very odd service to include in our discussion but, as we shall see, it is an excellent example that easily satisfies our definitions of telemedicine and telecare.

Approximately 10 years ago, a number of UK Local Authorities (LA) started to provide an emergency alarm system via the telephone for the residents of their properties in an effort to meet their obligations under the 'duty of care'. These systems have developed over the years in technical complexity, geographical coverage, and in the services provided.

When a large percentage of LA housing was transferred to private ownership, the operation of many, although not all, of these alarm services was also transferred to the private sector. Further details can be found in Fisk [200] and Thornton [201].

A community alarm service is a service offered to elderly people in nursing homes, warden-assisted residential homes and private dwellings, that allows them to communicate with a human operator at a remote call centre via a 'hands free' telephone. The service is available 24 hours per day and 365 days per year. Residents can initiate the call from anywhere in their home by use of a pendant alarm either located in an obvious position or worn like a brooch. The system automatically identifies the caller and displays the caller's details to the operator. The operator talks to the client, identifies what is wrong and then summons assistance as required.

About one million properties in the UK (and an estimated one and a quarter million people) are connected to a community alarm service. There are 350 call centres in the UK serving this community. Some services are small but others serve 40 000 clients spread over several locations. The small services tend to be run by the LAs whereas the larger services are privately run. The private services have often developed out of the private companies operating residential and warden-assisted homes developments.

There is obviously a minimum number of clients that makes a service economically viable and it is likely that many of the smaller services will be absorbed over the next few years to create a few (20 or 30) larger (private) services. This is beginning to happen now and has created a situation where clients in Merseyside and Harrogate (for example) are served by a call centre in Bath.

The community alarm service providers are looking to expand [202], not only by taking on more clients, but by offering more services. Some of the opportunities are:

- on-demand patient and carer information service;
- extension of the service to other groups like disabled clients, early hospital discharges and those needing palliative care;
- extension to conditions like AIDS/HIV, multiple sclerosis, epilepsy and diabetes;
- interactive systems in which the call centre checks on patients' functional status and relays information to the community healthcare team.

Clearly, the community alarm system in the UK has a well-established infrastructure that can be developed further for a large range of telemedical and telecare activities.

4.3.5   Non-Government Organisations

We should not end this section (or chapter) without mentioning briefly non-government organisations (NGOs), which not only respond to disasters of both human and natural creation throughout the world but which do such important work in developing countries (Section 1.5.2). NGOs are frequently charitable bodies funded by donations and, like managed care organisations, they need to engage in cost-effective activities to make their funds stretch as far as possible.

Telemedicine is a means to achieve this aim with the consequence that underdeveloped countries can sometimes find themselves using technologies, e.g. the Internet, ahead of citizens in more advanced countries. According to the World Health Organization [203]:

> remote diagnostic services, health education, the training of healthcare personnel, and the management of emergency situations are fields in which telematics has an increasingly important contribution to make.

WHO already has worldwide networks for the surveillance of the spread of drug resistance, pollution levels, and the adverse effects of pharmaceutical substances etc. International co-operation and funding are needed to bring the benefits of these knowledge bases to the populations who so desperately need them.

4.4 SUMMARY

In Chapter 4 we have seen that:

- We can currently identify three main ways in which GPs can use clinical telemedicine to benefit patients and themselves: monitoring of conditions, minor injuries and emergencies, and better coordination with secondary care.
- Acute hospital services use telemedicine to establish hospital–patient links, where patients are able to spend more time in their own homes, inter-hospital links, offering improved cover and specialist advice with support for practitioners in remote areas, and visual contact with patients to facilitate diagnosis and treatment.
- Telecare often has a social aspect to it, e.g. home visits by community nurses or midwives. Telemedicine can improve the efficiency of these visits, making some unnecessary and making time for others.
- Home healthcare is a rapidly growing segment of the healthcare market.
- Telemedicine can be used by ambulance paramedics to help the emergency room team assess the patient and buy valuable time before they arrive at the hospital.
- Pharmacists are only just beginning to consider the impact of telemedicine. The selling of prescription drugs on the Internet is highlighting a need for tougher controls.
- The main objective of managed care organisations is the delivery of high-quality and cost-effective healthcare. The major driver for both quality

enhancement and cost savings, however, is the reduction of use and stay in hospital and recuperation in the patient's home. Telecare is used to monitor patient's progress and recall the patient to hospital only if the symptoms demand it.

- There are two main thrusts in mobile telemedicine. The first is a strategic one: that is, to develop an organisational approach to dealing with events that can swing into action when these events occur. The second is the development of devices to extend the range of telemonitoring.

- Astro-telemedicine pioneers have carried out extensive research and development into biosensors and telemetry. They are now turning their attention to the miniaturisation of devices and their integration into health management systems.

- Military telemedicine has been more concerned with the treatment of physical injury and trauma. It is now looking to data warehouses to use the experience to detect disease or circumstances that could disable a fighting force.

- The community alarm system in the UK has a well-established infra-structure that can be developed further for a large range of telemedical and telecare activities.

- According to the World Health Organization, 'remote diagnostic services, health education, the training of healthcare personnel, and the management of emergency situations are fields in which telematics has an increasingly important contribution to make'.

5

DEVELOPMENT AND DELIVERY OF TELEMEDICINE SERVICES

OBJECTIVES

At the end of this chapter you should be able to:

- appreciate the importance of national healthcare policy on telemedicine development;
- compare the policy context of telemedicine in the USA, Australia, the UK and Malaysia;
- identify the local and the external policy drivers of telemedicine service development;
- understand the difficulties associated with evaluating telemedicine pilot studies;
- know how to assess needs when developing a telemedicine service;
- carry out the key stages in developing a telemedicine service;
- discuss the issues associated with the delivery of telemedicine services.

5.1 INTRODUCTION

By this point you should have a good idea of the scope, benefits and limitations, technology and applications of telemedicine. Chapter 5 attempts to put this knowledge to use and show you how to develop and deliver telemedicine services. The information gained will help you to participate in successful projects.

The chapter starts with a consideration of the national healthcare context in which a telemedicine project takes place since this context may well determine whether a project gets off the ground or not, or whether it succeeds or fails if it does start. Some countries, e.g. the USA, Australia, the UK and Malaysia, are developing national strategies for telemedicine and examples from their policy formulation are used to illustrate the importance of context.

The chapter continues with a look at the issues involved in evaluating pilot studies of telemedicine to see if they can be transformed into production services with definable healthcare benefits. This section addresses systems and services evaluation before tackling the more contentious issues of healthcare benefits and cost effectiveness.

Turning to the development of mainstream services, the steps needed to determine the viability of a telemedicine proposal—namely defining service goals, assessing needs and involving users—are all examined. We then proceed to study the design, development and delivery of the specified service. This stage looks at the generation of the business case, the re-engineering of existing practices, the establishment of practice guidelines and the management of the service.

5.2 THE STRATEGIC CONTEXT OF SERVICE DEVELOPMENT

5.2.1 The Roles of Government, Healthcare Professionals and Industry

In earlier chapters, we have considered the drivers of telemedicine (Section 1.4), the benefits it produces (Section 2.4) and the barriers to its development (Section 2.5). Government, healthcare professionals and industry all have roles to play [204] in harnessing the drivers to overcome the barriers and achieve the benefits. We will now examine these roles a little more closely.

The Role of Government

In a welfare system (e.g. the UK), the government is both the major (often monopolistic) purchaser and provider of healthcare for its citizens. In contrast, in a largely private-funded healthcare system (e.g. the USA) the government's role is mainly to produce a framework in which market forces operate. Whatever the system, however, all governments regulate healthcare by the laws they promulgate since these precepts determine the legal and (often) ethical environment in which healthcare professionals, managers and others function [205]. Governments also support healthcare by the priorities they establish and the developments they promote.

For example, irrespective of the healthcare system all governments must define laws to deal with data security, ethical standards of practice, liability and malpractice, fee payment, physician licensing and accreditation. The State will frame these laws in consultation with clinicians and other professionals but ultimately only parliament, congress or their equivalents can enforce them.

Similarly, if in its social programme an administration declares that improving the quality of life of elderly or disabled citizens, or extending healthcare to underprivileged communities, are priorities then it will facilitate the development of telemedical solutions to these problems. It may also promote solutions by introducing specific policies with underpinning funding. Indeed, when an issue becomes a component of governmental policy, then its very inclusion alters the perceived cost–benefit (if not the more objective cost effectiveness) equation since realising government objectives is itself a perceived benefit.

In the commercial sphere, the governments of all developed countries realise the importance of information and communications technologies (ICTs) for national competitiveness [206]. If they establish business environments that encourage investment, entrepreneurial activity and risk-taking then they will stimulate interest in new ICT application areas such as telemedicine and telecare. These policies will also open up new markets and export opportunities for telemedicine products and services.

These comments reveal the strength of the relationship between health and a nation's legal, social and economic frameworks. For telemedicine, they expose the importance of governmental policy and strategic direction setting since these actions dramatically encourage or inhibit developments.

Where policy is fragmented or underdeveloped, it is difficult for telemedicine initiatives to flourish. Thus, despite Japan's reputation as an integrated and technocratic country, the diffusion of telemedicine has fallen well below expectations [204, 207]. This failure is attributed to the conflicting objectives of local and central government, which hinder knowledge transfer and lead to a lack of coordination between government, users and manufacturers.

Healthcare Professionals

One important role of healthcare professionals in advancing healthcare standards and best practice has already been mentioned—the advice given to government to frame policy, legislation and guidelines. Clinicians and other healthcare professionals are uniquely qualified to provide this advice but by virtue of their claim of clinical autonomy they are also uniquely placed to block development if it counters their (usually status or financial) interests. Issues of licensure and reimbursement (see Chapter 6) therefore top the list of barriers to progress (Section 2.5).

In addition, the technological aspects of telemedicine and the intrinsic lack of direct, face-to-face contact with patients disturb some clinicians, who find such practices undermine the traditions they have been taught to value and believe are in the best interests of their patients [73].

In contrast, other practitioners have embraced telemedicine and the technology with enthusiasm. These individuals have a major role to play in working with their sponsors to research and create the circumstances in which telemedicine is a well-accepted adjunct or alternative to face-to-face consultation [208].

Finally, we recall that continuing medical education is closely linked to the practice of telemedicine. Healthcare professionals have an obligation to contribute to and avail themselves of the opportunities to improve their own skills and the medical services they deliver to their patients.

We see once again that the roles we have identified are discharged not in isolation but in collaboration with government and industry. This integrative approach is worthy of further comment and we return to it in Section 5.4.3.

The Role of Industry

Healthcare is the world's largest industry, accounting for 8% of the total world product [205]. Of this total, 15% is attributable to the mostly global pharmaceutical sector, 4% is due to medical equipment, and another 1.5% is credited to health information systems and technology systems, a sector dominated by a decreasing number of international companies. With its ability to deliver healthcare across national frontiers, telemedicine is poised to become a significant contributor to this industrial output.

The 'industry' we have in mind may be either a commercial enterprise operating in a free market, or a public body acting either as a monopoly or within a managed market. The industry may provide services or manufacture goods. In the USA, the telemedicine service providers are usually managed care organisations or hospitals associated with academic institutions. In the UK, the National Health Service is by far the major provider of services. In both countries, equipment manufacturers are commercial companies supplying their goods on the free market.

An important role of an industrial supplier (if they want to prosper) is to produce equipment that the purchaser wants to buy. In the telemedicine field this means mainly telecommunications products and infrastructure, or general-purpose videoconferencing equipment, perhaps modified to meet clinical requirements. Industry should therefore work with the legislature to establish telecommunications standards and to sell devices that conform to these standards.

Another function is to design and build hardware and software that are not only highly reliable but also easy to use. It is important that carers and patients involved in teleconsultations can concentrate on the healthcare issues and not need to respond to technical diversions. Authorities may assist requirements by issuing standards of accreditation that products have to satisfy before they are 'fit for purpose'.

The evolution of new products and ways of working presupposes investment in research and development (R&D) to exploit the latest technology and ideas. Companies need to support their customers with medium- and long-term strategies for product development that are nevertheless flexible enough to respond to scientific advances. Once again, the state can encourage R&D by tax breaks and other incentives.

But government may not be able to exercise its control as extensively and as exclusively as in the past. As business becomes more and more global, national frontiers begin to lose their significance and commentators speculate that multinational companies will start to act as quasi-governmental organisations [209]. Whether this happens or not, administrative policies friendly to business, and companies collaborating with healthcare professionals, are powerful partnerships to promote the development of telemedicine and telecare.

After this general overview of strategic issues, let us look at the frameworks adopted by various countries to facilitate the development of telemedicine.

5.2.2   The USA Context

The United States was an early player in the telemedicine and telecare field due to progress made in telecommunications infrastructure in the late 1980s and early 1990s. This facility has been matched by generous R&D funding by both federal and state agencies as well as by NASA. The US Department of Defense programmes have been some of the best-funded telemedicine programmes in the world. These high levels of support have given the USA its global lead in telemedicine.

The origins of the communications infrastructure can be traced back to the cold war period of the 1950s and 1960s with the introduction of the military's warning system, the Advanced Research Projects Agency Network (ARPANet) [22]. ARPANet eventually gave way to the National Science Foundation Network (NFSNET) serving the academic community until it too was replaced in 1995.

Perhaps the key development for telemedicine, however, was the creation of a high-speed national communications network mandated by President Bush in 1991 with the signing of the High Performance Computing Act (1991) [22]. When the Democrats came to power in 1992, Vice President Gore pronounced his vision of an information superhighway and the concept was translated into policy as the National Information Infrastructure (NII) [210] in 1994. NII identified telemedicine as a crucial health tool that would benefit from information technology [211].

The next significant advance was the Telecommunications Reform Act of 1996 [212], which was intended to increase competition among telephone providers, lower costs, and reduce regulation and bureaucracy.[1] Consumers are still apparently waiting for these benefits to become universally available.

As part of the NII initiative, a Joint Working Group on Telemedicine (JWGT) was formed with representatives from several agencies [211]. The Telecommunications Reform Act requires this Group to submit reports to

---

[1]   The Bill assumed a level of notoriety due to its infamous section 502, which outlawed the publication of obscene material on the Internet [212]. The clause was eventually defeated in a US Federal court by an action brought by the American Civil Liberties Union. The defeat was hailed as a victory for freedom of speech and pornography.

government summarising telemedicine activities as well as the results of federally funded studies. In this way, government is kept informed of progress in telemedicine and the need to facilitate it. See, for example, the 1999 Congressional telehealth briefing mentioned in Section 1.2.1.

In spite of the collaborative work of the JWGT much remains to be done to establish a strategic approach to telemedicine development. For example, in 1996, nine government agencies invested at least $229 million in telemedicine but there was no overall strategy to coordinate activity or maximise benefits. These deficiencies were highlighted in a General Accounting Office (GAO) report [213] in 1997 which recommended that the Department of Defense, responsible for over half the 1996 expenditure, should take the lead in devising a national strategy. Funding and information gathering continue.

The main issue is the usual one of reimbursement, although the GAO found no evidence to support the Health Care Financing Administration's assertion that offering fee-for-service reimbursement of telemedicine services to Medicare patients would vastly increase expenditure [214]. Since January 1999, Medicare reimbursement has been available for telemedicine services in rural counties [215]. Licensure and accreditation, malpractice and security issues are other common reasons for the slow progress.

One area in which progress is more visible, however, is the construction of practitioner guidelines. For example, the American Telemedicine Association has adopted a set of clinical guidelines for telecare, covering patients, health providers and technology [216]. An interdisciplinary group has also produced a report [217] on guidelines for telehealth practice for the JWGT as it develops recommendations for Federal and state legislative, regulatory and policy statements. This latter report is very comprehensive, covering standards of professional conduct and care, as well as clinical and technical standards, effectiveness and evaluation methodologies, confidentiality and documentation issues.

The USA is of course not alone in having a tension between national and state legislation and practice. What is needed, here as elsewhere, is a facilitating policy at national level that encourages knowledge creation and sharing [218] across state boundaries.

The setting of standards is an indicator that telemedicine is maturing and that healthcare professionals have sufficient experience to be comfortable with its application. In general, clinicians in the USA have enthused about telemedicine as a useful adjunct to conventional, face-to-face medicine and as a potential cost-saving tool. The greatest threats to physician acceptance take-up have been the reimbursement and other legal–ethical issues (again!) and the fear, expressed earlier [73], that the technology is too impersonal, not just in teleconsultations with the patient, but because it reduces informal 'what do you think?' sharing of information between clinicians. In spite of the potential, it seems there is still some way to go before telemedicine is just another way of practising medicine.

The same comment applies to commercial investment in telemedicine. One consulting firm predicts a $3 billion market by 2002 based on videoconferencing systems and teleradiology units [217]. Even so, the take-off point is still in the future, and HMOs and suppliers are wary of over-reaching themselves.

The main problems seem to be the low throughput and the high infrastructure costs. These factors explain why practitioners are turning more and more to less demanding store-and-forward applications and why teleradiology is so popular (together with insurers' willingness to reimburse this type of intervention). The USA has over 10 000 installed teleradiology units.

The most successful telemedicine providers are those that are active in conventional healthcare and have the critical mass and stability to diversify their operations [219]. Small, single-application start-up companies are more risky. To remain successful, however, all companies, whether service, product, or network suppliers, must continue to offer that most ethereal of commodities, 'added value'. This can take the form of complementary e-health services such as MRI or CT scans, or other services that overcome the remoteness aspect mentioned above.

Another, increasingly common, reason for venturing into remote medicine is the 'export' opportunity offering telemedicine services nationally or internationally. Some US academic institutions have been very successful in this way [219] while several managed care organisations have taken the view that if they do not do it, then the missed opportunity will become a threat as a competitor does it to them.

Finally, all players are looking forward to the day when telemedicine becomes a necessity, or at least a first choice, rather than an infrequent alternative to conventional medicine. This will be closer when telemedical practice becomes linked with the electronic patient record [219].

5.2.3 The Australian Context

Significant activity in telemedicine in Australia began in about 1991 and, as elsewhere, was mostly bottom-up, in this case spearheaded by healthcare organisations and companies at state level. In 1993, Crowe [220] published one of the first articles to raise more general issues and draw attention to the inevitable reimbursement and legal problems that present themselves wherever telemedicine captures attention.

John Mitchell of John Mitchell & Associates (Section 2.2.2 and references [4, 6]) appears on the scene about this time. His consultancy company was involved in several high-profile projects and Mitchell's evaluation reports on these projects endeavour to extract general principles and make recommendations for further developments (see, for example, the two surveys on South Australian projects to pilot telepsychiatry [221] and renal dialysis [222] that appeared in 1994 and 1995, respectively).

A more recent paper by Crowe [223] is also helpful in tracing the first attempts to provide telemedicine with a strategic dimension at Federal level. In 1996, the House of Representatives Standing Committee on Family and Community Affairs established an inquiry into health information management and telemedicine. This Committee, which published its *Health On Line*, report in late 1997 [224], received submissions on a wide range of issues, including feasibility, costs and benefits, standards and service implications. It expressed particular interest in rural applications, reflecting the vastness and remoteness of the Australian continent, and noted a lack of basic infrastructure on which to mount services.

1996 also saw the establishment of a working party of the Australian Health Ministers Advisory Council to examine a range of issues that needed to be resolved at national level. These issues were concerned with guidance on financing, inter-state registration of healthcare professionals, privacy and security, and equipment and reliability standards. Interestingly, criteria to evaluate projects were accorded a high priority [223].

More recently (1998/99), we have had the industry scoping study [4] and the report on e-health [6] commissioned by the Commonwealth Government from the Mitchell stable. We introduced and referred to these studies in previous sections. They are major reports intended as discussion documents to inform the strategy setting process. National workshops have been used to broadcast their message.

The executive summary of the e-health report recommends that everyone should work with everyone else to identify and solve the problems preventing telemedicine from entering mainstream healthcare. If this counsel seems a little obvious then the body of the report is more substantial, giving many case studies, an up-to-date list of telemedicine projects in Australia, and international comparisons to illustrate the 'unstoppable rise of e-health'. The range of projects demonstrates the willingness of healthcare professionals to embrace telemedicine, particularly in the many remote areas with which Australia is so well endowed.

The industry scoping study has a sharper focus and greater penetration. It concludes that most people see telemedicine as a mix of technologies, markets and customers, and few industry stakeholders have a clear picture of how information technology and telecommunications will impact on healthcare over the next few years. Some sections of the market (e.g. videoconferencing) are dominated by a few suppliers, thereby restricting competition. Enthusiasm and fascination with technology are no substitute for sound business planning and evaluation.

Other factors include the opportunities for exporting and selling healthcare, the limited infrastructure, the lack of dialogue and partnerships between vendors and buyers, as well as the usual financial, legal and cultural barriers to progress. Given the picture of uncertainty that the report paints, it is perhaps unsurprising that, while there is agreement that Australia needs a national coordinating body for telemedicine, there is no consensus as to what it should be doing. Should it concentrate on technology, promotion, evaluation, marketing or other issues?

The confused situation arises partly from the nature of a federation of states each wanting to preserve its autonomy.[2] However, the USA is also a federation, one where mistrust of central government knows no bounds, and national policy and strategy formulation are patently more advanced than in Australia. We simply observe that national strategy should be about establishing frameworks, incentives, directions and ground rules by which the various participants are encouraged to bring about the required changes.

5.2.4   The United Kingdom Context

Early work (1991 onwards) in the UK was concentrated in academic departments and in teaching hospitals. Its diffuse and exploratory nature focused largely on technology and proof-of-concept studies. There was little concern about how the studies could be scaled from pilot to production level and how telemedicine could enter the mainstream of the national health service. As a consequence, the national Information Management and Technology (IM&T) Strategy [225] launched in 1992 made no direct reference to telemedicine, although it did promote the idea of an NHS telecommunications infrastructure, NHSnet, which is now becoming a reality.

The need for a strategic planning framework began to be recognised in 1995 when the Department of Health commissioned a report on telemedicine activity within the UK [226, 227]. This survey confirmed the circumstances noted above. It found an awareness but little understanding of telemedicine. Activity (which consisted of 25–30 projects distributed around the UK[3]) was uncoordinated, and there were no comparative or cost-effectiveness studies.

The survey concluded that the introduction of telemedicine into mainstream medicine would not take place until the key issues were addressed. These issues were largely organisational but also connected with integrating telemedicine into healthcare policy and strategy.

The study was followed a year later by a similar review on telecare [228]. The results discovered 14 major telecare projects falling into three distinct categories: medical (outreach services from the secondary and tertiary sectors), technological (using communications to improve the quality of life of the elderly) and social (housing and social services organisations discharging their duty of care).

---

[2]   It was only in 1996 that rail travellers could for the first time go across Australia from east to west without changing carriages due to the different gauges of the state railways.
[3]   The up-to-date list of telemedicine projects is available at the Telemedicine Information Service web site [40] hosted by the University of Portsmouth.

The study showed that UK telecare lagged behind progress elsewhere except in one area, community alarm systems, where local authority and private initiatives demonstrated a powerful way of delivering care in the community. The report emphasised the need to build upon existing strengths via greater coordination between service providers and by the development of a broad economic model to define costs and benefits more carefully.

The recommendations inherent in these reports were eventually picked up at government level when the Labour government came to power at the 1997 general election. The modernisation plan for the NHS, *The New NHS* [36], made little direct reference to telemedicine, being concerned more with overall goals and the structural changes needed to achieve them. However, the way forward was hinted at in a section (para. 3.15) on the role of information technology to support quality and efficiency. These aims would be sought in several ways, including 'developing telemedicine to ensure specialist skills are available to all parts of the country'. The strategic role of telemedicine appeared to be to extend access to high-quality services.

This theme was developed within the new information strategy, *Information for Health* [37], published in 1998, which declared that 'opportunities in the field of telemedicine will be seized to remove distance from healthcare, to improve the quality of that care, and to help deliver new and integrated services' (para. 1.29). The integration of services was now a declared aim along with quality.

Information for Health is peppered with references to telemedicine and telecare, and at one point the document boldly proclaims (para. 5.5) that:

> Telemedicine and telecare will undoubtedly come to the fore as a way of providing services in the future. They have a key role to play in the Government's plans to modernise the NHS. Their development must be managed in a coordinated way, to ensure the benefits are properly identified and applied and scarce IT and other resources are not consumed ineffectively and inappropriately. An early priority will be a framework to guide the development and application of telemedicine and telecare.

Cost savings are now added to the equation and there is recognition that developments must be coordinated to achieve benefits.

More important than the rhetoric, however, is the requirement that local healthcare organisations 'routinely consider telemedicine and telecare options in all Health Improvement Programmes' thereby putting telemedicine on the agenda of every service planning authority. The same organisations were charged with formulating Local Information Strategies to realise the goals of *Information for Health*. Guidance on this process made it clear that 'The full benefit of telemedicine and telecare may only be realised in the light of managerial and organisational change' [229]. Culture, rather than technology, may be the rate-determining step.

The strategic vision articulated in these statements has got a little sidetracked by the high priority afforded to the NHS Direct telephone triage service [230]. However, it does seem that at Department of Health level there is a fundamentally sound appreciation of the issues associated with achieving the benefits of telemedicine and telecare within the National Health Service. Hopefully, the outcome will justify this confidence.

The UK does not suffer reimbursement issues to the same extent as countries such as the USA but the ethical and confidentiality aspects are equally compelling. It is therefore constructive that an academic institution, the University of Cardiff, has taken the initiative in setting up a Centre for the Legal and Ethical Aspects of Telemedicine [231].

One area where further thought is needed is the role of telemedicine equipment and service suppliers. Suppliers have in general been badly served by previous information strategies; for example, system specifications have often been stated without ensuring that any supplier can meet them. Real, sustainable progress will only be made if suppliers are involved in the planning of telemedicine developments.

5.2.5   The Malaysian Context

The three examples of telemedicine strategy development explored so far have all started with bottom-up, field projects followed by a realisation that a strategic framework is needed to maximise benefits. Malaysia is almost the complete reverse.

With clear vision and tremendous energy, Malaysia has embarked upon its intention to become a developed nation by 2020 (see Section 1.4.2). As part of this vision, in 1996 it launched the concept of the Multimedia Super Corridor (MSC) programme [38] with flagship programmes to revolutionalise government, business, education and health. The health programme, referred to simply as *Telemedicine Flagship Application* [39], uses the word telemedicine in a broader sense than the definitions we worked out in Chapter 1, but even this emphasis shows how the Malaysians see information and communication technologies as central to the delivery of all public services.

The vision is largely that of the very single-minded prime minister, Dr Mahathir Mohamed, who has driven the industrialisation and modernisation programme from the start. His leadership has been inspirational but his greatest contribution has been to encourage foreign direct investment into the country, particularly in manufacturing, financial services, and in the oil and gas industry. Economic goals have also been coupled with social targets to ensure long-term, sustainable growth with equity [232].

To encourage the essential investment, the government has drafted facilitating laws and established tax breaks and other financial incentives for foreign companies to set up business in Malaysia and to train and employ local workers. The high-tech Telemedicine Programme is a consortium of universities, government agencies (e.g. the Ministry of Health), medical service providers, healthcare financial organisations (e.g. managed care companies) and equipment suppliers. Like most MSC ventures, development is focused in the specially built region (the 'corridor') south of the capital, Kuala Lumpur.

The Telemedicine initiative emphasises 'wellness' by delivering seamless care and advice and empowering individuals to manage their own personal health. The four pilot applications to be developed over a five-year period and tested throughout the country for completion in 2010 are:

- *Mass Customised/Personalised Health Information and Education*: endeavours to deliver customised information on public health and individual conditions to the public at large.
- *Continuing Medical Education*: uses computing and communication technologies to help healthcare professionals update their knowledge and skills and offer the best services.
- *Teleconsultation*: will use multipoint technology to connect healthcare providers (patients are not mentioned) to share opinions.
- *Lifelong Health Plan*: the Malaysian equivalent of the UK's electronic health record to keep the individual in the best possible state of health.

This is a very ambitious plan that other countries are watching with interest [233]. Browsing the MSC literature, however, the reader is struck by the comprehensiveness and logic of the telemedicine strategy. It is refreshingly free of the clichéd political slogans and rhetoric which are almost *de rigeur* in government announcements within the UK. The core of the strategy, the partnership between the government, healthcare professionals and industry, and the accompanying incentives, sound right and seem set for success. We can only hope so.

5.2.6   General Principles of Strategy Development

We hope to have demonstrated the importance of a strategic framework in which telemedicine applications can flourish and enter the healthcare mainstream. We will finish this section by using our survey of some leading nations in the field to extract some general principles of strategy development. The principles apply to governments, healthcare providers and system suppliers. We will simply list them and let you spot any omissions. Here is the summary, which will also be helpful to us as we consider the development of telemedicine services in Section 5.4.

- Governments and other policy-making agencies should declare their purpose in seeking to promote telemedicine and telecare. Are the goals to improve quality of care, extend care to under-provided communities or to save money?

- Governments should facilitate the growth of telemedicine and telecare by establishing a framework of guidelines and regulations within which healthcare professionals and companies can work together. This framework should aim to facilitate, not control, developments.
- Governments should encourage partnerships between healthcare providers and commercial system suppliers by financial and other framework incentives.
- Governments, in partnership with healthcare professionals, need to address the legal and ethical issues accompanying telemedicine to ensure that these do not act as barriers to uptake.
- Excessive enthusiasm and overselling are recipes for disaster for telemedicine advocates, whether they are clinicians or suppliers.
- Vision must be accompanied by a sound business case and careful implementation.
- The business case should cater for future as well as current requirements.
- Telemedicine projects and services should focus on outcomes and manage participants' expectations.
- Telemedicine services should be offered as part of a portfolio of related services (not necessarily telemedical) or use shared infrastructures.
- Telemedicine services should integrate with existing services and, where possible, integrate healthcare holistically across sectors and agencies.
- Large organisations able to diversify from an established base in healthcare are more likely to succeed in telemedicine than small ones with specialised interests.
- An adequate volume[4] of teleconsultations or telemedical services is needed to show a return on investment.
- Telemedicine services can be exported into private healthcare and overseas markets.
- Alliances across sectors can stabilise developments (especially for small organisations) and can lead to valuable spin-offs, e.g. educational services.
- Education on service planning, development, implementation and operation is in itself a valuable service.
- Added value, e.g. the retention by clinicians of personal contacts or the offering of an additional out-of-hours service, are important differentiators of service.

Now that we understand the strategic context of telemedicine, we will turn our attention to how we can evaluate pilot studies of telemedicine to see if they can be transformed into mainstream production services with definable healthcare benefits.

---

[4] One review [234] found that only 12 programmes in the USA had performed more than 500 teleconsultations in 1997.

5.3 THE EVALUATION OF PILOT STUDIES

5.3.1 The Purpose and Scope of Evaluation

Evaluation has been a contentious issue in telemedicine development since the mid-1990s. Why is this? There are several reasons, reflecting fundamental uncertainties. For example:

- What are we evaluating?
- Why are we evaluating it?
- How should we carry out the evaluation?
- How should we interpret the results?

You can see the reasons for the uncertainty. Fortunately, an excellent chapter by Taylor [235] dispels much of the confusion. Taylor's chapter makes it clear that we are evaluating pilot studies of telemedicine and the purpose is to determine if they can be transformed into full-scale production programmes, i.e. into *mainstream* telemedicine.

We are not evaluating the mainstream programmes themselves. If we were, then we would define a range of *performance indicators* to determine how well the established programme meets its operational objectives and targets. We discuss this aspect in Section 5.4.8.

To answer the 'how should we carry out the evaluation?' question, Taylor distinguishes three areas of investigation:

- systems;
- service provision;
- healthcare effectiveness.

We shall look at each of these, drawing upon the expertise of Taylor and others as appropriate. However, there is one element of evaluation common to these areas that is worth considering separately. This fourth area for discussion is the *cost effectiveness* of telemedicine. We have referred throughout the book to the difficulty in demonstrating cost effectiveness (see, for example, Section 2.5) and we need to elaborate on the reasons why, and what we can do about it.

The final query in our list is 'how do we interpret the results?' and here, as we shall see, there is still a measure of ambiguity.

In considering our four areas we shall find they are underpinned by other fundamental characteristics, e.g. cost reduction, service integration, training etc., and we shall consider these from the various perspectives. These characteristics will surface again when we discuss the development and delivery of a full telemedicine service in Section 5.4. We give cross-references where appropriate.

5.3.2   Evaluating Telemedicine Systems

The main goal of systems evaluation is to ensure that the healthcare data provided by telemedicine are as useful as those provided by conventional means. Taylor [235] describes this task as 'establishing the safety of telemedicine'. The goal needs elaboration. First, to be 'useful' the data must have certain attributes. For a start, they must be relevant, accurate, current, complete and consistent. Then they must be accessible, so that we can retrieve information (useful data) at will, and manageable, so that we can extract details and interpret them to draw conclusions.

Second, in requiring the data to be 'as useful' as data from conventional means, we are tacitly acknowledging that data utility (quality) is not an absolute entity with a gold standard attached to it. Instead, data quality is a relative concept and we judge it by comparing it with some reference standard (e.g. data quality obtained by conventional means) that we find acceptable for our purpose.

To test the utility of telemedicine information we should carry out experiments under controlled conditions comparing data from the telemedical and non-telemedical interventions. If the studies involve actual patients then ideally the same patients should be seen in both studies.

In effect, the data we obtain from these studies are the outcomes of the experiments. The variables that determine these outcomes depend upon the technical system features and the medical condition under investigation. Thus, telecommunications bandwidth might be a strong determinant of quality with a real-time telepsychiatry application but less so with store-and-forward teleradiology. Other technical features of importance include image display (resolution and colour integrity), camera quality, ergonomics and ambient lighting [236]. These and other factors are described in Chapter 3 and the references therein.

Equally important in determining data quality and system safety are the procedures and guidelines laid down to conduct interventions. We met process guidelines in Section 2.3.2 and these protocols, together with clinical guidelines and care pathways, determine the progress of a teleconsultation and the data collected. Telemedicine and conventional studies will necessarily have different guidelines.

There may be other, unavoidable, differences between telemedicine and control studies that affect the interpretation of the data from the two experiments. One critical factor is the often unfamiliar nature of the telemedical equipment and procedures to the healthcare professionals involved in the study. Clinician training is therefore a vital prerequisite if valid comparisons are to be made. Section 5.4 returns to this issue.

Many other factors can confuse the interpretation of the results and the conclusions drawn. For example, radiologists claim to be able to detect subtle lesions on X-ray films that are absent on digital monitors used in teleradiology.

However, Gale *et al.* [237] found that major discrepancies between telemedicine and conventional interpretations occurred in 1.5% of cases compared with 0.96% disagreement using purely conventional means. Does this mean that teleradiology is inferior to conventional radiological examination? If the use of teleradiology meant that you could provide a screening service for patients who would otherwise get no treatment at all would you deny the service on the grounds that it was a substandard technique?

Similarly, Gerbert *et al.* [238] studied the abilities of GPs and specialists to diagnose skin problems. The GPs failed to diagnose malignant melanomas by conventional means 40% of the time, compared with the dermatologists, who were in error 26% of the time. Neither success rate is particularly good but the results surely suggest that a telemedical link to a GP practice giving online access to a remote dermatologist would be a safer procedure than leaving the GP to his or her own devices. This conclusion is supported by the education and skilling opportunities offered by the link for the GP, who may quickly achieve the same success rate as the specialist.

The message of these comments and examples is that 'like-with-like' comparisons are very difficult to achieve. The decision about the viability of a telemedicine proposal may well depend upon a whole raft of factors, clinical, economic, technical (and political), some of which may be well beyond the control of those participants. Section 5.4 looks at these factors in more detail.

5.3.3   Evaluating Service Provision

Service provision issues are mostly logistical or connected with training [235]. Thus, a frequent cry heard from clinicians is 'we would use the system more if it was available when we wanted it'. Scheduling equipment availability at both ends of the remote link and matching it with clinician availability is no mean task, particularly when there are competing uses for the facilities [239]. Even when equipment and clinicians are available, it may still be tricky to get the patients to the remote site—a difficulty experienced with one prison inmate study [240] in the USA. Patients with more free time may still find getting transport to the remote site difficult and telemedical appointments are just as susceptible to 'don't shows' as are their more traditional counterparts.

Patient satisfaction with a telemedicine service is usually determined by questionnaires but these must be devised professionally if they are to be valid reflections of opinion rather than a self-fulfilling exercise. Even then, patients are notably less concerned with the suitability of the service than with the quality of the healthcare intervention. This observation may indicate that the service is no worse, and is probably better, than the equivalent they receive by conventional means. However, hard, scientific evidence on comparative service provision is clearly difficult to come by.

An evaluation framework developed by the American Institute of Medicine contains useful examples of questions put to patients and carers on ease of access and their perceptions of the quality of telemedicine services [241]. We say more about the design and delivery of production services in Section 5.4.

The training needed to use telemedicine equipment, and acquisition of the experience to maximise the benefits, are considerable overheads that may be very unattractive to clinicians not convinced of the merits of the technology. Like any other skill, the clinician's initial exposure must be reinforced by practice and by further learning to achieve the same level of expertise that he or she would bring to conventional treatment. Add to this the need to master unfamiliar technology and deal with unforeseen technical problems and it is scarcely surprising that some clinicians prefer the familiar ways.

Mitchell's report on the Queensland Telemental Health Programme contains some helpful observations of the content and organisation of training sessions [242]. An important feature of the training for this project was that staff were coached in interview and communication skills as well as in technical competence. The preliminary evaluation attributed much of the success of the project to this combination of skills, which increased the clinicians' confidence and ability to use the systems effectively.

5.3.4 Evaluating healthcare effectiveness

Although service quality and healthcare quality are closely connected in a consultation, our interest here is to see if we can isolate and evaluate the latter features, i.e. the clinical effectiveness of the telemedical intervention.

If the telemedicine study is concerned with the refinement of an existing process of healthcare, then the evaluation is likely to concentrate on the process itself and how it has changed. Where telemedicine is used to provide a new or different type of service, however, we tend to focus on outcomes rather than processes [235]. So which outcomes do we measure? As with systems evaluation, that depends upon the nature of the study. If the intention is to reach new communities then the number of patients presenting from these communities in a given (short) time is clearly an important measure of success. If we want to know if telemedicine can help us to diagnose a potentially terminal condition at an early, more treatable stage then survival rate is an important outcome and we may (hopefully) have to wait some time to interpret the data.

Patient satisfaction with the healthcare aspects of a teleconsultation is as important as their concerns about logistical arrangements. Patients will feel comfortable with the teleconsultation if they can see and hear clearly during the interview process and they are assured of its confidentiality. They must also be convinced that the video and audio systems are transferring the information needed for the consultant to come to a reliable assessment of their condition.

It is when patients are asked to compare telemedicine and conventional treatment that the difficulties arise. By its very nature, a pilot study often requires special working arrangements and patients may express a preference for telemedicine simply because they are getting a better service, e.g. less travel, shorter waiting times etc., rather than a better medical outcome [243]. Again, patients are really not in a position to judge the relative quality of diagnosis or treatment by different methods [244].

The accepted way to separate these effects is by randomised control trials (RCTs). RCTs have been used to demonstrate health improvements in patients with hypertension [65] and diabetes [66] who have checked their condition by using telemonitoring devices at home (could the improvement have something to do with the convenience of being at home?). Recently, some doubt has been voiced about the applicability of RCTs in health technology assessment where new technologies are undergoing rapid change as the trial progresses [245, 246].

Interestingly, despite the above examples, there have been comparatively few attempts to show that telemedicine actually improves patients' health and most of these have been unsuccessful [235].

Reference [241] identifies some interesting questions that can be used to evaluate quality of care and health outcomes. These questions compare telemedicine and conventional treatment and include:

- differences in the quality, amount or type of information available to patients and carers;
- differences in patients' knowledge of their health status and understanding of care options;
- differences in diagnostic accuracy or timeliness;
- differences in health-related behaviour, e.g. drug compliance;
- differences in morbidity or mortality;
- the immediate, intermediate and long-term effects of the telemedicine treatment.

5.3.5   Evaluating Cost Effectiveness

The cost effectiveness of telemedicine has become a *cause célèbre* over the past few years [247–249]. There are several reasons for this interest. First, as already made clear, initial studies of telemedicine were mainly grant funded and concerned more with 'proof of concept' and technical aspects than demonstrating cost effectiveness. It is also no accident that some of the major project funders were (and still are) space and military agencies, who view cost effectiveness differently from civil agencies. Once telemedical interventions were shown to be practicable, however, workers in the field began to realise that the new techniques would never win general acceptance unless they were seen to be cost effective compared with alternative methods.

Second, it is difficult to devise a funding model for telemedicine that allocates costs accurately. Remote working is not restricted to a range of medical conditions untreated by other techniques. It should complement and integrate with existing methods and share resources, making it hard to separate costs. Pilot study costs can also be quite different from production costs where economies of scale are apparent and existing services and practices are modified [89]. Simple activity statistics for telemedicine will not reveal these effects.

Third, even with an acceptable funding model, researchers have struggled to demonstrate cost savings in telemedicine pilots partly because the studies have been so small. Finally, as also pointed out, telemedicine has proved remarkably resilient to attempts to prove its effectiveness, i.e. clinical worth, compared with conventional techniques. This is partly due to the difficulty in quantifying (and costing) intangible benefits, e.g. the reduced isolation of rural physicians [250] or the multiple uses of shared telecommunication links [251].

This catalogue of reasons has presented a formidable challenge and researchers have risen to the occasion to such an extent that some pioneers have suggested that telemedicine can be over-evaluated [89]. Yellowless [90, 91] in his principles for successfully developing a telemedicine system states principle 6 as 'Telemedicine applications should be evaluated in a clinically appropriate and user-friendly manner'. In this context the word 'appropriate' means testing if the outcomes defined in the business plan (Section 5.4.4) have been achieved within an agreed timescale and resource allocation and to the required level of quality. In effect, Yellowless is saying that cost-effectiveness evaluations of pilot studies are of limited use.

In Section 1.4.2, we referred to the article by Allen and Stein [35] that gives a detailed account of cost effectiveness across a range of telemedicine applications. Their assertion that general teleradiology, telepsychiatry, and home and prison telecare (telemonitoring) are most likely to be cost effective is backed up by many of the examples they quote. However, the authors' descriptions and comments underline the uncertain nature of several of the claimed cost savings, both in terms of costs underestimated or ignored and the benefits, for which costs cannot easily be assigned.

Rather than quote uncertain statistics, we will draw your attention to two studies that have proposed frameworks for the evaluation of telemedicine. The first (1997) by McIntosh and Cairns [252] is concerned mainly with economic evaluation. The paper describes the economic issues and the main challenges to evaluation, and then goes on to advance a set of evaluative questions that formally link costs and consequences. This is an attempt not only to identify the key issues in telemedicine evaluation, but to adopt a more holistic approach than the usual concentration on the short-term implications of a well-defined part of the overall process [235].

The authors list the main difficulties facing economic evaluation as:

- constantly changing technology (see reference [245]);
- lack of appropriate study design to manage small samples;

- inappropriateness of conventional techniques of economic evaluation;
- the valuation of health and non-health outcomes.

A more recent (1999) paper by Hailey *et al.* [253] suggests a more generalised evaluation framework and applies it to a specific telepsychiatry service in Canada. The framework includes five elements: specification, performance indicators, outcomes, summary measures, and operational and other considerations. Interestingly, application of the framework to the cited study showed that telemedicine presented no cost benefits to the service provider but it was much cheaper for the patient. It is difficult to know if this conclusion would extrapolate to other studies.

It appears that we have still some way to go in our attempts to find a suitable framework for evaluating cost effectiveness let alone in showing that telemedicine is cost effective. Perhaps the advice of Yellowless and his principle 6 is the most pragmatic and useful after all. Perhaps, as Mitchell [254] suggests, telemedicine will become part of e-health and we shall all wonder what the fuss was about. The ultimate test will be when some large US managed care organisations take the plunge and demonstrate conclusively that they are making money out of telemedicine. Then we shall wonder why we didn't believe in cost effectiveness before!

Fortunately, the snares and pitfalls of evaluation have not deterred the more adventurous souls from developing and running telemedicine services and we can now turn to see how this is done.

5.4 DEVELOPING AND DELIVERING A TELEMEDICINE SERVICE

5.4.1 Defining Service Goals

In Section 1.4 we discussed the technological and non-technological factors that have driven the development of telemedicine and telecare and have raised their profile with policy makers, healthcare providers and commercial enterprises. With increased awareness of the technical and service options, these agencies are better placed to design, plan and implement mainstream telemedicine services to ensure their success. But how do you build a telemedicine programme (see reference [255] for one answer)?

The first step is to define the service goals. What is the project trying to achieve and is telemedicine the best way to deliver the objectives? As we have seen, telemedicine can be a bit of a technological 'honey-pot', attracting participants who are intrigued by the novelty and reputation-making nature of remote techniques. Self-deception is always a risk in these circumstances and it is bad policy to support a proposal simply because the technology looks interesting.

Careful and objective analysis is needed to determine the real motives for a project [256]. The reasons for going ahead might still be motivated by political priorities but they must involve healthcare professionals and potential users and be clinically sound. From our previous discussion, telemedicine is liable to be a strong choice when the main service goals are:

- improved quality of care;
- extended access to care;
- cost reduction;
- better collaboration and integration;
- educational opportunities.

The telemedicine proposals most likely to succeed will satisfy several of these goals. A key factor in these deliberations is the nature and extent of existing services. For example, a prime candidate for telemedical support is a service that is routinely referred out of district or region [257], most commonly due to the lack of the trained personnel.

If, following this qualitative analysis, telemedicine looks as if it is the appropriate technology for the project, then it becomes necessary to quantify the needs of the target population [258]. Only then can we decide if the service can meet these needs and be sustainable within the imposed constraints.

5.4.2   The Assessment of Needs

For simplicity, we can confine ourselves to three types of need—clinical, economic and technical—and consider each of these in turn. Further information on needs assessment is provided by Doolittle and Cook [256].

Clinical Needs

Clinical needs can be defined in several ways but the following criteria are especially important:

- *Nature of specialty.* We have seen (Section 4.2.2) that certain specialties, i.e. those that require external, visual examination, are well suited to telemedicine. If the patient's condition lends itself to such examination then telemedicine may well meet the clinical need. If not, e.g. if the condition demands an internal examination or surgical intervention, then more conventional, face-to-face methods may be necessary. Telemedicine may still meet part of the clinical need.
- *Purpose of service.* The needs, and so design and cost, of the service will differ depending on whether the main purpose is communication between physicians or the diagnosis, monitoring or treatment of patients. For

example, a diagnostic cancer service will have fewer resource demands than one that offers treatment involving chemotherapy. This will be especially so if the remote carer is unfamiliar with the treatment and uncomfortable with providing the service at a distance from the specialist.

- *Personnel and training.* Following on the previous point, meeting a clinical need may require additional personnel or a training requirement, especially at the remote site if healthcare professionals are unfamiliar with the equipment and its operation. These demands may impose unacceptable overheads on the project, which, if they cannot be met, may reduce its scope or cause it to be abandoned since it would be unsafe to proceed.

- *Service integration.* When considering clinical need it may be possible to use telemedicine to improve the integration of services (see also Section 5.4.3). Thus, a minor injuries centre could transmit X-rays to a physio-therapist working in a primary care practice, or a GP could share case notes on a psychiatric patient with a social care worker. These extensions constitute 'added value' and need not be particularly expensive.

Economic Needs

We can similarly define a few simple criteria for the evaluation of economic needs. All of these criteria are influenced by the volume of teleconsultations. Estimates of the levels for each type of activity are essential to the assessment of costs and income.

- *Staff.* The staff of a new telemedicine service may be new appointments or personnel recruited from existing staff. Either way there is a cost implication which must be factored into the assessment of economic needs. While doctors, specialists and nurses are the most obvious appointments, the non-clinical requirements should also be considered. The latter will certainly include technicians to support the running and development of the service, and possibly clerical staff and office managers. Again, costs can be reduced if existing staff are willing to undergo career-enhancing training and undertake new roles, particularly if additional remuneration is on offer.

- *Capital and revenue costs.* Capital costs are usually associated with tele-consultation equipment, network infrastructure and facilities such as buildings. They are obviously important in the start-up phase but will re-occur if and when the service is upgraded, especially if the revised service demands greater bandwidth. Decisions need to be made on how these costs are apportioned between the various participants, for example between a hub and its remote sites. These decisions can be made on purely economic grounds, e.g. a remote centre may incur line costs if it makes extensive use of a network connection or have these costs offset if it brings in a significant number or reimbursable referrals to the specialist centre. Alternatively, costs can be distributed according to some policy formula. often appropriate if the project is sponsored by a grant or charitable foundation.

- *Income and reimbursement.* The distribution of earned income should be addressed at the needs assessment or design stage since any delay can lead to friction, which can nullify the benefits of the service. Each circumstance is different, as the previous criterion on costs demonstrates, and it is important that all principals are involved in the decisions. Physician reimbursement is a different problem and negotiation with funding agencies or insurers may be necessary to determine the economic viability of the service.

- *Reorganisation costs.* Telemedicine services can cause considerable upheaval for carers, not least if they reduce or replace existing services. If the service is based on a hub and several remote centres, the departmental reorganisation at the hub is the most common disturbance with considerable cost implications. Costs may also be incurred by relocation of other services to group telemedicine staff and equipment together and streamline delivery.

- *Patient-incurred costs.* Patients may incur additional costs such as travel, time off work and child care, and these should be included in the assessment.

Technical Needs

Criteria for the assessment of technical needs include technology audit, network infrastructure, and user requirements.

- *Technology audit.* The technology audit identifies not only the equipment that must be purchased to run the service but, since these requirements are often modest, existing equipment, e.g. videoconferencing systems, which can be pressed into service. The type of equipment needed will depend on the nature of the service. For example, a desktop unit is appropriate [256] for many clinical purposes but a rollabout system is better for videoconferencing or medical education where group interaction is needed. Some patient conditions will also require specialised telemonitoring equipment which may have limited use outside the telemedical service. All equipment should be easy for non-technical people to use.

- *Network infrastructure.* The network infrastructure may be owned and under the control of the telemedicine team but it is more likely to be leased from and maintained by a telecommunications provider. In this case, it is certain to present a cost overhead that cannot be avoided. In addition, a successful service will create a demand for higher bandwidths and the technical need may translate into an economic one. Flexible bandwidth configuration is highly desirable, as are alliances to share infrastructure and costs.

- *User requirements*. New technology can be daunting to both patients and carers, and it is important to assess their needs so that they feel comfortable with the equipment and procedures. This requirement may have a cost implication but it is unlikely to be high and well worth paying to ensure acceptance and satisfaction with the service. Similarly, frequent users may have preferences for the type of equipment that is specified, e.g. the distinction between rollabout and desktop systems noted above. Or technicians may prefer a certain type of equipment or technology because it is easier to maintain. These and related issues should be assessed by involving users, patients and suppliers in the specification of requirements and the purchasing decisions.

5.4.3   User Involvement

It is evident from what we have said already that user involvement is an essential component of telemedicine development. By users we mean both carers and patients. These are the front-line people who will largely determine the success or failure of the service. Their expertise and experience is vital to ensure that the service is not only goal-driven but rewarding to use. From their ranks will come the 'champions' whose enthusiasm will lead the developments and push them through against inevitable setbacks.

It is also vital to have the commitment of senior clinicians and managers, who should be visible supporters of the project at all times even if they are not directly involved in detail developments.

Let us build upon our needs assessment to summarise some of the more important aspects of user involvement. Other issues are conveniently dealt with in the articles by Yellowless [89–91] referred to in Section 2.4.2 and picked up in later sections.

- *Involve remote sites*. Our previous comments echo Yellowless' Rule 1 [89] and Principle 2 [91] that users should own the system. In the excitement and rush of planning it is only too easy to develop a centralist approach and underestimate the importance of users at the remote sites—typically the *raison d'être* for the service. These users, both carers and patients, should be involved in the design and operation of *their* site.
- *Manage user expectations*. The expectations of users are important not only in designing a service but in monitoring and improving it. Users with little experience of healthcare delivery let alone telemedicine are often daunted by procedures that carers may feel are trivial, and patients can readily be put at ease by simple explanations of what is going to happen to them and what the outcomes and timescales are likely to be. Long-standing patients switching from traditional to telemedical treatment come with expectations which condition their acceptance [259] of the new

technology, and learning from these experiences is a powerful way to deliver best practice.

- *Build teams.* The service will be most successful if the individuals identified in the needs assessment process see themselves as members of a team. Clinicians, nurses, technicians and administrators (and patients) may well have different perspectives on the development and operation of the link, and team building is the necessary process of combining these multi-disciplinary outlooks into a coherent approach. Recognising the validity of other people's views and acknowledging their efforts (publicly wherever possible) are essential to this process. It is also possible that a team at a remote site has a different approach to another at the central location. Reconciling these different attitudes and mindsets may be an additional challenge [256].

- *Ensure training.* Whatever the expertise among the project leaders there will be significant need for technical and clinical-related training among the team members. A plan for initial and ongoing training (as people leave and join) is essential for the well-being of both staff and patients. It may well be worth involving selected patients in this plan since they can act as strong advocates of the service.

- *Locate services.* The needs assessment stage will identify priorities in terms of clinical need, and planners may be tempted to site link points within areas of highest concern. However, clinical needs must be balanced against economic and technical needs and it is wisest to locate link points where user involvement and expertise are highest. See Yellowless' Rule 3 [89].

- *Integrate services.* Needs assessment and team building may identify opportunities for service integration, for example, using a telemedicine link to facilitate patient monitoring in the community after a teleconsultation or a discharge from hospital. Another, more ambitious option, might be a disease management programme (see Section 4.3.1 and reference [187]). Cross-discipline user involvement is the key to integrated service development, and planners should be proactive in harnessing these opportunities.

- *Market services.* External marketing (not over-selling) is essential to ensure the take-up and growth of the service. Internal marketing and information sharing among healthcare colleagues via seminars, workshops and evaluations is also necessary to promote the service and avail the participants of constructive criticism. Again, it may be helpful to encourage past and future patients to take part in these ventures.

5.4.4   The Business Case and Planning

Although they are ongoing exercises, needs assessment and user involvement are essential elements of the business case to attract funding for a telemedicine project and for planning its implementation. What else goes into the case depends upon the local circumstances and what the planners learn in these processes. However, based on our discussion so far, we can identify certain core elements that should appear in every case (see [89–91, 214, 217] for further information). Clyburn [260] presents a highly detailed analysis of the business case for telemedicine in terms of business process reengineering (see Section 5.4.5), change management and organisational culture. Although interesting, the pragmatic approach adopted here is more relevant to most practitioners.

- *Define the real objectives.* As we have seen (Section 5.4.1 and reference [256]), 'pseudo' objectives are sometimes offered to give credibility to a project case which is really nothing more than a bid for funding techno-enthusiasts to experiment with technology. This is unfortunately most common with academic grant submissions. The outcomes of such awards may solve useful problems but not necessarily those for which the grant was awarded. To win support and trust in the telemedicine world the project must seek one or more of the service goals noted in Section 5.4.1, to which we can add efficiency and revenue generation. The business case should make clear whether the proposal is a pilot or a full production project.
- *Define population and demand.* For telemedicine to enter mainstream medicine it must be sustainable by a critical mass of teleconsultations and/ or other activities (e.g. medical education). The business case is therefore more likely to succeed if it can demonstrate (realistic) benefits to a large section of the public or to some vulnerable section of it, e.g. children. A project may also capture attention if it addresses often terminal conditions such as cancer, multiple sclerosis or HIV/AIDS that have no routinely effective cure. Finally, a case may be funded for political as well as clinical reasons if it reduces a significant deficiency in service provision, for example the UK waiting lists for surgical operations.
- *Show the connection with existing services.* We introduced this point in our discussion of needs assessment. A mainstream role for telemedicine will only come about if the approach can integrate with vital existing services. Where there is conflict with existing services, the business case should describe the impact of the new telemedicine system, how it might make some services (and staff, particularly consultants) redundant and extend others. Everyone can be a winner if the case can show savings in facilities and the release of personnel who can be employed in other understaffed areas of the organisation. Finally, it is worth bearing in mind that the chances of success, in both winning support and achieving objectives, are more certain if the project deals with telemedicine services that have been successful elsewhere.
- *Summarise technical options.* The business case is no place to rehearse detailed technical arguments. However, since the case must state the financial implications, it is wise to explain technical choices in the broadest

terms so that those evaluating the case recognise that they are getting value for money. Value for money might equate to low cost but 'fitness for purpose' is a more convincing argument. Both the business case and the subsequent planning should demonstrate how the service will use the equipment and network to its full capacity, if not straight away at least over a defined period. Projects that specify expensive technology and then underuse it are unlikely to receive continued support. The business case should also plan for the future, and flexibility and expandability often carry their own cost. Evaluators will recognise the merit of paying the extra if the arguments are clearly put.

- *Describe the benefits.* This is an obvious section of the business case elaborating on the service goals of Section 5.3.1. The case should also highlight any added-value components implicit in the service goals. For example, patients could be directed to Internet resources and support groups for their condition, or a telecardiology service could be linked to wellness programmes for healthy diet and exercise.

- *Consider alliances.* As suggested in the discussion on technical needs, alliances with other organisations are useful for sharing expensive resources such as medical equipment and network infrastructure. Where the partners have complementary skills and facilities, such an alliance can extend the services beyond what either could offer and gain a competitive edge or unique selling point. However advantageous technically, some alliances may be politically sensitive and these are best avoided—at least in the business case.

- *Indicate market opportunities.* The removal of the distance constraint on care delivery opens up several possibilities for the more entrepreneurial-minded clinician or health services manager. Examples include:

  - opportunities for consultants to use telemedicine to practise overseas;
  - possible use of civil telemedicine facilities by military organisations;
  - health support contracts with transport organisations, e.g. airlines, shipping;
  - opportunities for telemedicine consultancy and education;
  - opportunities for private sector referrals or new fee-based convenience services.

- *Project management.* The business case should show how the project to plan and implement the service will be managed. A good project management methodology such as PRINCE [261] is a critical requirement given the diverse cultures of the participants and their geographical distribution. PRINCE offers particular benefits via its focus on outcomes and the provision for rigorous risk assessment and contingency plans. For a start-up project, the business case should request funding for an experienced, full-time project manager who can drive the project and ensure the service is introduced on time, on budget, and to the required (and expected) quality levels.

5.4.5 Business Process Reengineering

Business process reengineering (BPR) [262] implies an attempt to break down an organisation's business practices into their component parts and re-assemble them to form a new machine. Traditional, large organisations operate on the 'Adam Smith principle' (*The Wealth of Nations*, 1776), by which economies of scale are obtained by training groups of workers to contribute specialist skills efficiently to the manufacture of products or delivery of services.

BPR challenges this dictum. It uses information technology as a catalyst to reengineer so that a smaller number of non-specialists can handle the whole process. It examines the whole organisation, or that part of it under scrutiny, to see which processes are essential, which can be improved, and which can be cut out without real loss. Planning, execution and control, decision making, workflow and reporting; all are taken apart and reassembled, making IT an integral part of the new operation.

Telemedicine is a new way (process) to deliver medical care and it relies heavily on information technology. It follows that the introduction of tele-medicine into a healthcare organisation should give many opportunities for BPR to increase quality and efficiency and lower cost. Interestingly, there are very few reports of its application to telemedicine, largely due, perhaps, to the cultural differences between healthcare and the business world.

Given the potential of both BPR and telemedicine, this is a pity, as the only substantial article [260] relating the two topics demonstrates. In contrast, here are just a few examples by which reengineering of conventional care through telemedicine can bring benefits:

- reduction in travel for patients;
- closer collaboration of clinicians in primary and secondary care;
- availability of international medical expertise in real time;
- improved clinical and administrative workflow [263];
- seamless integration of care services across sectors;
- use of telemedical monitoring devices in the home.

These examples reveal that in practice, the introduction of telemedicine nearly always involves BPR although it is often as a consequence of 'introducing telemedicine' rather than a proactive attempt to discover opportunities for streamlining services and increasing efficiency. A more proactive BPR approach could pay considerable dividends.

5.4.6 Selecting the Technology

Technology underpins the successful delivery of telemedicine but it is not an end in itself. Chapter 3 describes the main technology components of a telemedicine system, e.g. videoconferencing stations, display systems, tele-monitoring devices, telecommunication options etc., and relates them to the applications and clinical procedures for which they are suitable. Familiarity with the content of this chapter will help a service planner to answer most of the essential questions or refer them to experts and suppliers. For convenience, we simply list some of the technology issues associated with the design and development of telemedicine systems (see also the technical needs discussion in Section 5.4.2):

- the bandwidth needed to deliver the necessary service effectively;
- the network infrastructure and its installation and maintenance;
- appropriateness of hardware and software for store-and-forward or real-time operation;
- conformance of equipment with accepted standards;
- the choice of videoconferencing station, e.g. rollabout, desktop etc.;
- the display definition and colour depth of the display [264];
- the need for and use of telemonitoring devices;
- the need for fault-tolerant and back-up systems;
- the need for date and time stamping for audit purposes;
- security and confidentiality requirements;
- user acceptance of technology;
- impact on the organisation.

References [265, 266] describe extended studies of technology assessment in telemedicine, including the acceptance, adoption, evaluation and implications of its introduction.

5.4.7   Establishing Practice Guidelines

Teleconsultations, especially those involving patients, must follow appropriate guidelines. In Section 2.3.2 we illustrated the format of a typical process guideline written as a checklist of the sequence of steps encountered in the consultation process. Here, we are concerned not so much with a clinical checklist or protocol but with how we design *practice guidelines* [217] to ensure an effective, safe and high-quality telemedicine service.

We should also reiterate the distinction between guidelines and regulations. Unlike a regulation, a guideline is not binding upon the practising healthcare workers. It is a digest of perceived good practice, which may not seek completeness. In particular circumstances the practitioners may therefore depart from it if they judge that the divergence is in the interest of the patient.

Let us look at some of the generic criteria for validating guidelines and their purpose. Naturally, a specific guideline must be written for every procedure but the criteria are valid for all cases. References [45, 72, 267] are good sources of further information.

- *Purpose of the teleconsultation.* In Section 2.3.2, stage 1 of the checklist was to 'explain the purpose and process to the patient'. In the context of validation, however, the guideline needs to make clear the overall aim of the teleconsultation, i.e. whether it is diagnosis, treatment or the monitoring of a condition (see Section 5.4.2). This requirement is necessary because the resources needed for the different procedures may differ widely. The guideline should therefore state the teleconsultation and medical equipment needed so that the clinician in charge can verify that the necessary resources are available.
- *Definition of responsibilities.* In traditional procedures, responsibility for the patient's treatment and well-being lies with the clinician who is in charge of the intervention at that time. This person may be the patient's GP or consultant, or a surgeon but he or she is always a qualified doctor licensed to practise medicine (and perhaps telemedicine [267, 268]) in the location where the intervention takes place. In telemedicine procedures, there is scope for ambiguity since there may be two clinicians involved, a GP with the patient and a specialist at the other end of the remote link. Alternatively, there may be a nurse or another healthcare professional with the patient who may act to some extent as a proxy for the remote specialist. The guideline must therefore make clear the competencies required of the various participants. It should also specify that these must be established, and the necessary authorisations received, before the teleconsultation can proceed [74].
- *Ensuring an ethical basis.* Normal rules of patient confidentiality and security apply to the storage and transmission of patient data derived from telemedicine. Data may only be transmitted with the informed consent of the patient and only data relevant to the patient's condition and problem can be sent. These constraints are essential to preserve the patient–doctor relationship and the autonomy of the patient. For these reasons, the guideline should require that the doctor and patient can reliably identify one another at the start of a teleconsultation.
- *Ensuring quality of care.* We have already noted (Section 5.2.1) that participants in a teleconsultation must be satisfied that the technical standard of the equipment and its operation, safety and security are fit for the intended purpose. These quality considerations must also apply to the collection of data and to the documentation of the whole consultation just as they would to a traditional patient–doctor interaction. Healthcare professionals at both ends of the telemedicine link may contribute to the record of the consultation and the notes should identify the authors of these contributions.

While the benefits associated with guidelines are highly desirable, they are not easy to achieve. Some of the most commonly cited limitations include the difficulty of getting the layout right and pitching the content at the right level [269], the threat to professional status, the perceived restrictions on good

practice [270] (change the guideline!), and the legal implications of a documented guideline that was not followed or that encouraged unsound practice
[271] (see also Section 2.4.2).

5.4.8   Implementing and Managing the Service

Telemedicine is a new way of delivering medicine. Consequently, its implementation will therefore disturb and even disrupt existing practices. Planned
and sensitive change management is therefore central to the successful
introduction of a telemedicine service. Other critical success factors include the
organisation of hub and remote sites, data collection and performance
indicators, and development plans. We will look briefly at each of these factors.

- *Managing change.* The world is knee-deep in literature on change management, much of it less inspiring that the trees from which the paper was
  made. There are nevertheless some useful theories and recommendations
  [272, 273] for effecting change. Key issues involve:
  - understanding the present;
  - setting goals and objectives;
  - leadership;
  - people involvement and communication;
  - overcoming resistance to change;
  - keeping up the momentum.

  Perhaps one of the most useful sources is Rosabeth Moss Kanter's book,
  The Change Masters [273]. Her keen sense of the value of the individual as a
  contributor to a team, and her insight into why it is easier to introduce
  change into integrative (team-based) as opposed to segmented (hierarchical)
  organisations are valuable lessons for would-be telemedicine implementers.
  We have highlighted the importance of teams (at hub *and* remote sites) and
  champions, as well as the incremental rather than 'big bang' approach
  (Section 3.5.1) to change management. Mitchell [222], in his evaluation of
  the renal telemedicine project at the Queen Elizabeth Hospital, Adelaide,
  adds system ease of use, training, goals, good organisation and documentation as other contributors to success. Warisse [274] has studied the
  changes in communication processes that organisations experience as they
  implement new communication techniques.
- *Organisation of hub and remote site.* Pursuing the above points (and those
  made in Section 5.3.3), implementers should ensure smooth arrangements
  for scheduling telemedicine sessions, and for reliability, security, documentation and technical support at all sites. Equal importance attaches to
  the integration of the new telemedicine services with existing services to
  encourage their move into mainstream activity [275]. System changes and
  interruptions should be advised well in advance of the events and carried

out outside of normal service times wherever possible. This is all good systems administration (and common sense) but it emphasises credibility and encourages clinicians to use the facilities.

- *Data collection and performance indicators.* The clinical results of teleconsultations and systems operation data relating to these sessions underpin quality assurance of the care process. The same data are crucial for setting performance indicators and checking the achievement of targets. Essential data should therefore be collected on a routine basis and used to build an expanding database that allows managers to measure performance and instigate improvements. Here are some examples of operational data that define useful targets for this purpose:
  - numbers of patients seen (including gender, age, ethnicity and social status);
  - percentage of correct diagnoses via telemedical link;
  - numbers of patients with successful medical outcomes compared with conventional care;
  - travel time and costs for patients to attend teleconsultations;
  - patient satisfaction with the service;
  - number of patient complaints;
  - operational system hours;
  - length of each teleconsultation or other session;
  - out-of-hours usage;
  - item and total costs compared with budget allocations;
  - amount of income generated.

Demographic data such as names of participants and the identities of the connected sites should also be recorded.

- *Development plans.* A successful service will lead to further developments, and managers should be aware of new opportunities. These might take the form of added-value inducements to use services, the expansion of existing services, or the addition of new ones such as treatment of new conditions or extension to other geographical areas. These improvements can even be packaged together, for example, by offering international, fee-based services to companies with employees on overseas business or to airlines or shipping organisations. In planning such developments, managers should take into account the impact on existing (including non-telemedical) services and the likely effect of increased demand on system bandwidth.

5.5 SUMMARY

In Chapter 5 we have seen that:

- Government, healthcare professionals and industry all have roles to play in setting the strategic context for the development of telemedicine.

- Governments should facilitate the growth of telemedicine and telecare by establishing a framework of guidelines and regulations within which healthcare professionals and companies can work together. This framework should aim to facilitate, not control, developments.
- An important role of healthcare professionals in advancing telemedicine is to advise government on policy, legislation, guidelines and best practice. Clinicians and other healthcare professionals are uniquely qualified to provide this advice but by virtue of their claim of clinical autonomy they are also uniquely placed to block development if it counters their interests. Issues of licensure and reimbursement therefore top the list of barriers to progress.
- An important role of an industrial supplier is to produce equipment that is easy to use and the purchaser wants to buy. Industry should therefore work with healthcare professionals and with the legislature to establish telecommunications and other standards and to sell devices that conform to these standards.
- The United States was an early player in the telemedicine and telecare field due to progress made in telecommunications infrastructure in the late 1980s and early 1990s. However, much remains to be done to establish a strategic approach for telemedicine development.
- Australia and the United Kingdom are similarly placed with bottom-up developments but little overall strategy to promote telemedicine. Australian strategic thinking seems rather confused at present but the UK government appears to understand that it must take a lead.
- Unlike these countries, Malaysia has defined a strategy before embarking upon many pilot projects and is establishing a framework to encourage industry to spearhead developments.
- The evaluation of telemedicine pilot studies is fraught by questions about why, what and how to carry out the evaluation and how to interpret the results. Four evaluation areas can be distinguished: systems, service provision, healthcare effectiveness and cost effectiveness.
- Key conclusions from these studies show that 'like-with-like' comparisons are very difficult, service provision issues are mostly logistical or connected with training, patients' comparisons of telemedicine and conventional medicine treatment are unreliable, and it is not easy to demonstrate either healthcare effectiveness or cost effectiveness.
- Defining service goals, assessing needs and involving users are essential steps in the development and implementation of a mainstream telemedicine service.
- The business case defining outcomes and performance indicators is also central to success. Other key aspects are the selection of technology, the establishment of practice guidelines and the management of the service.
- Service planners should look proactively at how business reengineering principles can be applied to existing practices when introducing a telemedicine service.

- Change management techniques can help the introduction of telemedicine especially if they emphasise team-based organisation and careful organisation at both hub and remote sites.

6

ETHICAL AND LEGAL ASPECTS OF TELEMEDICINE

OBJECTIVES

At the end of this chapter you should be able to:

- discuss the telemedicine implications for patient confidentiality, rights and consent;
- comment upon the doctor–patient relationship in telemedicine;
- analyse the issues surrounding access to medical records;
- interpret the role of data protection and security legislation;
- identify the concerns associated with electronic data transmission;
- describe the circumstances of telemedical malpractice and clinical negligence;
- describe approaches to minimise the occurrence of malpractice complaints;
- appreciate the impact of licensure and reimbursement on telemedicine development;
- understand the implications of intellectual property rights for telemedicine.

6.1 INTRODUCTION

In previous chapters, we have traced the origins and development of telemedicine, its benefits and limitations, the technology used, who are the main users, and how we can develop and deliver telemedical services. This is quite a journey and you should have gained many insights into the potential impact of telemedicine on healthcare delivery.

You will also have noted frequent comments throughout the text on the ethical and legal issues associated with the new technologies and the concerns that they produce. This last chapter is devoted to a survey of these issues. It will not delve into great detail since it is not a treatise on morality or law but it will try to expose the important elements and their impact.

We start with the concepts of confidentiality and patient rights and consent. We review the doctor–patient relationship, consent to treatment and the disclosure of information, as well as access to medical records. The legal framework of data protection and security is next on the agenda, leading to some practical aspects of secure access and transmission.

Then we turn our attention to telemedicine malpractice, what constitutes duty of care and clinical negligence, and how the medical profession is both endeavouring to safeguard patients and reduce its own exposure to litigation. The thorny issues of clinician licensure and reimbursement are also discussed.

Finally, we take a look at intellectual property rights and how they are used to encourage innovation and protect the reputation of telemedicine products and services. Our constant companion throughout this survey is Stanberry's book [11], which is referred to on numerous occasions.

6.2   CONFIDENTIALITY, PATIENT RIGHTS AND CONSENT

6.2.1   Confidentiality and the Law

The principle of confidentiality in medical ethics dates back to Hippocrates. It has been developed in various codes, including the International Code of Medical Ethics [276], which states that a doctor must preserve 'absolute confidentiality in all he knows about his patient' even after the patient's death. But does this code of practice, however venerable, have a foundation in law?

In the United Kingdom, the legal perspective of confidentiality has its origins in the fields of contract, equity and property law [27]. As a consequence, it has evolved gradually on the basis of precedence and case law and represents pragmatic solutions to current problems rather than a framework of comprehensive and integrated principles. It also focuses on the relationships between the persons involved rather than the systems by which they communicate. The latter systems are dealt with by data protection legislation, as we shall see in Section 6.3.

The guiding principle behind this legal perspective is the concept that information is held to be confidential if its release has the potential to injure a person either emotionally or materially. This concept applies whether or not a contract or other formal relationship exists between the confider and the confidant. Confidence is not betrayed, however, if what is disclosed is common knowledge or if disclosure serves a greater public interest.[1]

Various health-related enquiries and reviews have sought to build upon this principle and develop it to recognise changes in the way healthcare is delivered. For example, in the UK, the Caldicott Committee's *Report on the Review of Patient—Identifiable Information* [277, 278] noted the 'information

---

[1] It is of course this latter exception which is the declared reason behind the many sordid 'revelations' that appear in British tabloid newspapers.

explosion' as introducing new risks for confidentiality. Fresh risks arose from developments such as seamless care, evidence-based medicine and organisational development as major drivers of change.

Irrespective of their legal systems, most democratic countries now base their modern practice of patient confidentiality [267, 277, 279] on the following three guidelines [267]:

- There exists a basic right of patients to privacy of their medical information and records.
- Patients' privacy should be observed unless waived in a meaningful way (i.e. informed, non-coercive) or in rare instances where it counters public interest.
- Information disclosed should be limited to that information or portion of the medical record needed to fulfil the immediate and specific purpose.

The legal force of these and additional guidelines may differ not only from country to country, but in federal nations such as the USA, from state to state. US Federal legislation to standardise state laws and the practice of telemedicine across state borders is still in the process of development [280].

Naturally, the guidelines apply to all forms of information. However, as we shall see, telemedicine creates special problems due to the involvement of non-clinical personnel in teleconsultations (Section 6.2.2), and the vulnerability of transmission lines to security breaches (Section 6.3).

Most of what we have said so far applies to patient-identifiable information, i.e. information that can be used to identify the individual it applies to. The legislation and guidelines do not apply to anonymised information stripped of any attributes that can identify the owner. This simple distinction between the two types of information is apparently not so clear-cut in practice. Thus, the British Medical Association's confidentiality rules were recently branded as unlawful by the UK watchdog Association of Community Health Councils [281]. The dispute centred on the collection and sale of data on doctor's prescribing habits and the difficulty of anonymising patient information completely, making it possible to identify patients and their medical conditions.

Guarding the privacy and confidentiality of health information is clearly an international concern in the global information society [277, 282, 283] but with this background we can begin to explore the confidentiality issues raised by telemedicine.

6.2.2   The Patient–Doctor Relationship

The duty of confidence lies at the heart of the patient–doctor relationship. Patients who reveal personal information to their doctors must be able to trust them not to divulge the same information to others incidental to the care process. The UK General Medical Council's (GMC) guidelines [284] on the duties of a doctor summarise international opinion by stating that:

Patients have a right to expect that you will not disclose any personal information which you learn during the course of your professional duties unless they give permission. Without assurances about confidentiality patients may be reluctant to give doctors the information they need in order to provide good care.

The GMC Guidelines make no distinction between conventional face-to-face medicine and telemedicine consultations and, as indicated, this duty is not absolute and can be overruled if disclosure is compelled by law or is in the greater public interest. However, by its nature, the practice of telemedicine raises more opportunities for confidentiality breaches and damage to the patient–doctor relationship than are apparent with conventional medicine.

For example, the duty of confidence applies to all information given to a teleconsulting doctor by a third party. If this party is a healthcare professional with close proximity to the doctor then they will be aware of the special nature of the patient–doctor relationship and acknowledge that they are under the same obligation of confidentiality. What, however, if the third party is remote from the patient, possibly in another country, or is not a healthcare professional at all but perhaps a technician working with clinical staff to ensure the quality of a radiological image and its error-free transmission?

In this case, the duty of confidence still lies with the clinician in charge of the consultation [27], but the third-party participants may not be fully aware of the ethical aspects of the patient–doctor relationship and may unknowingly or otherwise betray this confidence. Patients may therefore become uncomfortable with the involvement of third-party persons in teleconsultations (particularly when these persons are at the other end of the telemedical link) and may refuse to participate or feel reticent about providing valuable information. Recognising this problem, the American Medical Association has begun to develop guidelines [267] for the supervision of non-physician providers in telemedical practice.

The involvement of individuals who are exposed to confidential information but who do not feel bound by the same duty of confidence as the consulting doctor underscores the vulnerability of the telemedical process. Another, almost self-evident, source of vulnerability is the requirement to transmit information electronically between consulting sites. The networks over which transmission occurs are susceptible to taps or offer the opportunity for hackers to access databases and other confidential information at hub and remote sites.

The secrecy requirement applies to the full range of transmitted information—text, data, images, video and audio—whether this information is generated within the teleconsultation itself or obtained from other sources such as medical records. Encryption can be used to reduce the likelihood of breaches and digital signatures can be used to authenticate messages and ensure that they have not been tampered with during transmission. We look at these technical controls in Section 6.3.

Many of the confidentiality issues arising in telemedicine can be addressed by a common-sense application of existing medical guidelines. However, the above examples show that there are telemedicine aspects that need special consideration. Certainly, there is a requirement on the designers of teleconsultation systems to ensure that these systems comply with accepted ethical practice and preserve rather than compromise the bond of trust between patient and doctor.

6.2.3   Patient Consent to Disclosure of Information

The previous section illustrates the central importance that both patients and doctors place on the privacy of patients and their right to confidentiality. Most patients accept, however, that their treatment will be undertaken not by one person, the (tele)-GP or (tele)consultant, but by a multidisciplinary team. They understand, therefore, that the principal physician in charge of their case will need to ensure that all members of the team have the information necessary to discharge fully their professional roles in the care process.

Once again, the GMC guidelines to doctors [284] make the points clearly. Following the statement noted previously, they continue by declaring that:

- When patients give consent to disclosure of information about them, you must make sure that they understand what will be disclosed, the reasons for disclosure and the likely circumstances;
- You must make sure that patients are informed whenever information about them is likely to be disclosed to others involved in their health care, and that they have the opportunity to withhold information;
- You must respect requests by patients that information should not be disclosed to third parties, save in exceptional circumstances (for example, when the health or safety of others would otherwise be at serious risk);
- If you disclose information you should release only as much information as is necessary for the purpose;
- You must make sure that health workers to whom you disclose information understand that it is given to them in confidence which they must respect;
- If you decide to disclose confidential information, you must be prepared to explain and justify your decision.

These guidelines make plain the responsibilities of the clinician in charge of treatment and the members of his or her care team.

Because of the clear need to inform members of the care team, the law assumes the implicit assent of the patient to the disclosure of information to them. In English law, written consent by the patient for this purpose is therefore not only unnecessary but irrelevant, although medical authorities may wish to obtain it as a safeguard.

Telemedicine offers a circumstance in which this precaution may be useful, i.e. the situation noted in the previous section where a third party who is not a healthcare professional receives personal information that can be used to damage the patient. However, it is by no means certain that patient consent would prevent a healthcare professional or his or her employers from facing prosecution for failing to provide a duty of confidence.

In most other circumstances beyond the care process, the patient's explicit consent is required to disclose identifiable health information. This consent is normally obtained in writing. Examples include permission to release information for research purposes, or to make public a medical condition where the risk of infection is slight but further controllable by putting the information in the public domain.

A final point concerns the circumstances in which a patient's refusal to disclosure can be overridden by the doctor or other authorities [27]. These circumstances arise when a patient's medical condition poses a serious threat to the community at large. An example occurs when a traveller has a notifiable disease such a cholera or plague. Telemedicine may then have a useful role as an aid to diagnosis or as a telecommunications link to advise immigration authorities of the danger. Other examples arise when a patient is mentally unstable and liable to inflict injury on innocent people, or when a doctor is obliged in law to assist in the investigation of a serious crime or misdemeanour, committed or merely contemplated.

In general, however, telemedicine is no more prone to these circumstances than conventional medicine.

6.2.4   Access to Medical Records

If a patient consents to disclosure of personal health information then he or she has an obvious interest in knowing what information is recorded in their medical record. Obtusely, in many countries the duty of confidentiality discussed in Section 6.2.2 has been manipulated by clinicians to prevent patients from gaining access to this information. The reasons offered for this denial have ranged from unprofessional practice to the inability of patients to understand the information recorded on their records. It was commonly held that clinicians 'owned' the records, were under no obligation to release details, and in any case were working for the 'patient's own good'.[2] There were

---

[2]   Most property law assumes that the owner of an item of property has that item in their possession or leases or licences it for the use of some other person(s) under a contractual arrangement enforceable in the courts. In this way the owner exercises control over his or her property. In the absence of a legal agreement, English common law assumes that the person who controls the use of an item is the person who creates it. Since the clinician is the person who 'creates' the medical record in its physical or electronic form, common law supports the view that the clinician or the health organisation for which he or she works is the 'owner' of the record. This view, long held in the UK, has been contradicted by the Access to Medical Reports Act 1988 and Access to Health Records Act 1990 as described in the text.

whisperings that the refusal to release information conveniently hid errors of medical judgement but by and large the public trusted the doctors and accepted that they 'knew best'.

All of this has changed with the rise of consumerism in the 1980s. The emphasis on consumer rights now encourages patients to claim access to their medical history and doctors to respond positively to these requests. In the UK, and in other developed countries [280], these changes have exposed the anomalous position of medical records with regard to ownership and control. Confidential details in the records originate with patients but the records themselves and access to them are traditionally controlled by clinicians acting on behalf of healthcare organisations.

Current thinking tends towards (but has not yet reached) a division of ownership in which the healthcare organisation 'owns' the physical record and the patient 'owns' the information contained within. Clinicians, by virtue of the trust placed in them by the patient, can access the information in the record for the benefit of the patient but they cannot, except under special circumstances, deny the patient access to the medical information.

The development of this position can be observed from two pieces of legislation introduced between 1988 and 1990 [27]. The first piece, the Access to Medical Reports Act (1988), gives patients limited rights to control reports created for employment or insurance purposes. The employer or insurer must obtain the patient's consent to disclosure prior to seeking a medical report on their status. The patient may consent to this request unconditionally or on the condition that they have access to the report. The conditions of this Act are relevant to the potential use of telemedicine to provide occupational health services. Disclosure of confidential patient information to an employer may carry risks for the patient whereas non-disclosure may carry risks for the patient's fellow workers. In addition, a teleconsulting doctor is obliged to draw a company's attention to conditions that may adversely affect the health of his (tele)patients.

The second piece of legislation is the Access to Health Records Act (1990). This Act gives patients access to health records made after 1 November 1991 and to earlier information if it is needed to make sense of the later information. Patients do not need to make formal application to exercise their rights although patient access outside the scope of the Act is subject to the doctor's discretion. The main grounds for exercising discretion, and possibly denying access, are when the doctor believes that the information is deleterious to the patient's health or when release of the information could jeopardise the confidentiality of other persons. Both circumstances are conceivable in telemedicine.

Although, medical records legislation in the UK is still underdeveloped, it does not suffer (for the moment at least) the sometimes confusing and contradictory legislation that afflicts the United States [280]. Here the lack of Federal legislation leaves state policy makers to enact confidentiality and access laws on a local basis even though telemedicine permits the transfer of medical records across state boundaries outside the providers' and legislators' control.

Concern over these issues has led to the passage of a Medical Records Confidentiality Act (1995) (S.1360) [285] and further developments are in the pipeline. Those interested in the broad scope of confidentiality and electronic records in the USA should refer to a National Library of Medicine publication offering a comprehensive bibliography of articles dealing with the confidentiality of electronic health data for the period 1990–1996 [286].

6.2.5   Consent to Treatment

Every competent adult has a right to refuse or consent to available medical treatment or healthcare. Thus, the clinicians in charge of this care must obtain a patient's consent before proceeding with the treatment. Any clinician who proceeds without this consent runs the risk of prosecution for tort of battery or negligence.[3]

The purpose of consent is twofold [27]. There is a clinical purpose which recognises that the cooperation of the patient is an important factor in the efficacy of treatment, and a legal purpose protecting the carers against a criminal charge of assault or battery, or a claim for damages for trespass to the person, or negligence. The legal protection is necessary if carers are to treat patients without fear of reprisal from individuals who later regretted their agreement to medical intervention.

Courts will only accept consent as a valid declaration if patients are made fully aware of the options available to them so that they can make an informed choice. Consent may be implicit (e.g. offering an arm for a blood pressure measurement) or explicit (e.g. signing a form of consent before a surgical operation). In all cases, however, those responsible for the treatment must ensure that the patient understands the implications of their decision and in particular that they are prepared to accept the medical consequences if they reject a form of proposed treatment.

The GMC guidelines [284] on the duties of a doctor state the position clearly by requiring doctors to:

> give patients the information they ask for or need about their condition, its treatment and prognosis; give information to patients in a way they can understand; [and] respect the rights of patients to be fully involved in discussions about care.

---

[3] A tort is an act which causes harm to a person or corporation, whether intentionally or not. It is a breach of a duty arising out of a personal relationship which is either contrary to law or an omission of a specific legal duty. In the UK, courts dealing with patient consent to treatment have moved away from tort, which implies intrusion (battery) upon the patient's rights, in favour of negligence, implying inadequacy of information on which to give or refuse consent.

As we have noted already, the ethical aspects of telemedicine are similar in many respects to conventional medicine but telemedical practice sometimes leads to more testing situations. Consider, for example, a merchant seaman or NATO soldier who needs telemedical advice or treatment but his medical officer, immediate shipmates or military colleagues do not speak his native language. Or what should be done if a holiday-maker not able to understand fully the language of the country he or she is in requires rapid treatment in a remote community? What do you do if the patient and doctor speak the same language but the medical condition requires emergency treatment and there is a videoconferencing link but no audio? What if the teleconsultant cannot speak to the patient directly but has to communicate through another physician?

These and similar conundrums raise further issues regarding patient consent to treatment. First, the GMC guidelines state the amount of information that the patient is entitled to on ethical grounds, but how much does the law require? The famous test in English law is the Bolam test [27, 287], which proscribes 'as much detail as a recognised body of medical opinion considers appropriate'. What the lawyers want to avoid here is making authorities on issues that have no unique interpretation. This may be reasonable although it clearly creates scope (intentionally?) for much argument and litigation. What is perhaps surprising in this age of consumerism is the reliance on a body of medical experts who might be expected to close ranks when one of their number is under attack. Perhaps this will change in the wake of recent events.

A second difficulty, highly relevant to telemedicine, is the point at which a patient should be asked to give consent. A company might provide telemedical cover for their employees who have to travel to remote areas on company business. Should the company require their staff to agree to accept treatment as part of their contract of employment? Neither the company nor its employees can foresee all of the circumstances in which consent would be required and it is always possible that an employee might want to change their decision. Blanket consent of this sort may be convenient for commercial organisations but it is inconsistent with current medical ethics.

At the other end of the spectrum, consent is obtained at the start of a programme of treatment. This has the advantage that the details of the consent closely match the treatment but of course it may not be possible to obtain the required consent in an emergency—again, this is particularly relevant to the telemedical treatment of travellers. In these circumstances, clinicians are legally bound to perform interventions deemed essential to safeguard life and health unless there is strong evidence that the patient would have withheld consent for religious (e.g. blood transfusions refused by Jehovah's Witnesses) or other reasons.

In such emergencies, or where the patient is otherwise incapable of giving consent, doctors often seek a 'proxy' consent from a relative, and a telemedical link may be useful in this context. However, legal opinion in the UK and USA tends rather to favour a temporary or 'quasi-proxy' status conferred on the physician in charge of treatment and to whom the patient is assumed to devolve his or her decision making.

A third and final problem noted here arises when a patient refuses treatment. For example, a patient may be willing to receive treatment but only by conventional means and not by telemedicine. Alternatively, and reflecting the global nature of modern medicine, telemedical treatment may be acceptable but not by certain practitioners, e.g. an Albanian patient might not wish to be treated by a Serbian doctor. Yet again, a patient may refuse treatment on moral or religious grounds (see above).

In these situations, patients with the capacity to do so are required to sign a written record stating the fact of their refusal and accepting its medical consequences. These records are usually generated by the healthcare provider but there is no reason why they cannot be drafted by the patient, as happens with Jehovah's Witnesses.

Clearly, these and other examples create difficult ethical dilemmas for doctors. However, provided the doctors have taken all reasonable steps to confirm consent, and there are no issues of negligence, then the legal framework is usually sufficient to defend them from prosecutions brought by patients who may feel that they have been unjustly treated (or not treated).

6.3   DATA PROTECTION AND SECURITY

In Section 6.2.1, we pointed out that the legal perspective of confidentiality focuses on the relationships between the persons involved rather than the systems by which they communicate. We must now turn our attention to these latter systems and data protection legislation. In the earlier section, we pointed out that telemedicine shared many features of confidentiality with conventional medicine. However, telemedicine's use of telecommunications to deliver healthcare raises particular issues of data security that we need to consider.

In the UK, there are three primary pieces of legislation relevant to our discussion:

- The UK Data Protection Act (1984)
- The UK Computer Misuse Act (1990)
- The UK Data Protection Act (1998)

We shall consider the general and telemedicine implications of each of these Acts although we need not repeat those aspects dealing with individual access to personal data (medical records).

6.3.1   The UK Data Protection Act (1984)

For over 15 years the UK Data Protection Act (1984) has regulated the use of automatically processed information relating to individuals, and the conduct of services in receipt of such information [287, 288]. The Act requires the registration of individuals and organisations, including NHS Trusts and health authorities, that hold personal information on computers, as well as bureaux that provide services to personal data users. There are criminal penalties for failing to register and for acting beyond the scope of the registration. The Act allows individuals to find out who holds information on them and what the data contain, as well as obliging organisations to disclose their activities.

Schedule 1 of the Act lays out the eight data protection principles.

1. *The information to be contained in personal data shall be obtained, and personal data shall be processed, fairly and lawfully*
2. *Personal data shall be held only for one or more specified and lawful purposes*
3. *Personal data held for any purpose or purposes shall not be used or disclosed in any manner incompatible with that purpose or those purposes*
4. *Personal data held for any purpose or purposes shall be adequate, relevant and not excessive in relation to that purpose or those purposes*
5. *Personal data shall be accurate and where necessary kept up to date*
6. *Personal data held for any purpose or purposes shall not be kept for longer than is necessary for that purpose or those purposes*
7. *An individual shall be entitled:*
   (a). *At reasonable intervals and without undue delay or expense:*
      - *To be informed by any data user whether he holds personal data of which that individual is a subject; and*
      - *Access to any such data held by the data user; and*
   (b). *Where appropriate, to have such data corrected or erased*
8. *Appropriate security measures shall be taken against unauthorised access to, or alteration, disclosure or destruction of, personal data and against accidental loss or destruction of personal data*

Principle 3 deals with disclosure of patient-identifiable data, and principles 4, 5 and 6 apply to the collection of data for patient records and the transmission of those records in telemedical applications. Principle 7 describes the patient's entitlement to access and principle 8 places the healthcare organisation under a responsibility to secure data against interference. Appropriate security measures include anonymising identifiable data wherever possible, encryption (see Section 6.3.5), secure entry to rooms and system authorisation.

The 1984 Act applies only to the automatic (i.e. by computer) processing of personal (i.e. person identifiable) data [287]. The Act defines 'processing' widely to mean adding, deleting or editing data or extracting data, including sorting data by subject. Note that an organisation could check how many telepatients it had without invoking the provisions of the Act provided the patients were not identifiable from the output. Also, word processing is excluded from the Act.

There are several exemptions to the Act covering such issues as national security, payroll and accounts, use by private individuals and clubs, examination marks etc. Healthcare organisations can withhold data from patients if disclosure would harm the patient mentally or physically (Section 6.2.4). They must also specify to whom they will disclose information in normal operation, e.g. the healthcare workers associated with the patient's care, and not release information to anyone else.

Stanberry's book [287] gives full details of the Act and European equivalents and alternatives.

6.3.2   The UK Computer Misuse Act (1990)

In the UK, the Wireless Telegraphy Act 1949 and the Interception of Communications Act 1985 offer civil and criminal remedies against the interference of telemedicine data during electronic transmission [287]. The Computer Misuse Act (1990) was introduced to provide protection against the misuse of data held on stand-alone or networked computers.

The Act was introduced as a private member's bill and came into force on 29 August 1990. The provisions are broad and aimed at combating various forms of misuse such as hacking, unauthorised access, illegal copying etc.

Three new offences were created under the Act.

1.   unauthorised access to computer material;
2.   unauthorised access with intent to facilitate commission of further offences;
3.   unauthorised modification of computer material.

A person is guilty of an offence if:

- he causes a computer to perform any function with intent to secure access to any program or data held in any computer;
- the access or intended access is unauthorised;
- he knows at the time when he causes the computer to perform that function that this is the case.

Most computer crime is perpetrated either by dissatisfied employees or by hackers. The former are intent upon malicious damage whereas the latter are usually concerned more with the intellectual challenge of gaining access to prohibited systems. However, both categories of abuse can cause serious damage and disruption. For example:

- confidential records can be read, copied, or erased;
- records may be changed;
- viruses may be introduced to cause immediate or delayed havoc.

Specific sections of the Act (4–9) contain provisions relating to computer crimes committed from outside the UK, or committed from within the UK and causing harm in another country. These provisions are particularly relevant to telemedicine.

The new law was designed to avoid tangible evidence difficulties that had arisen in the 1980s. The Act does not provide a complete answer to problems of unauthorised access to computers and few cases have been brought to the courts. Perceived problems include:

- organisations are often reluctant to bring cases of hacking and virus penetration to court because of bad publicity;
- the police have difficulty collecting evidence;
- telecommunications companies are not obliged to reveal information;
- mainframe computers cannot be retained as evidence—the police have to rely on local expertise and advice as to what material can be collected as evidence;
- files can be erased without trace;
- juries appear to view hackers (and perhaps virus spreaders) as maverick 'Robin Hood' characters pitting their wits against the 'system';
- sentences are perceived as being too light in comparison with the seriousness of the offences;
- judges and barristers/advocates lack the specialist knowledge of computers to apply the law as it was intended—they tend to make inappropriate interpretations.

These criticisms support the thesis that computer crime is a fast-developing field and that legislation needs updating to reflect the opportunities available to both criminals and officers of the law.

6.3.3   The UK Data Protection Act (1998)

The European Directive on Data Protection was agreed in 1995 and became law in October 1998. Its provisions were incorporated in UK law on 1 March 2000. The Data Protection Act (1984) meets many of the requirements of the new law, which extends the earlier provisions in the following significant respects [287]:

- it defines key concepts differently;
- it extends data protection controls to certain manual records;
- it sets more stringent conditions for processing personal data;
- it affords certain exemptions for the media;
- it strengthens the rights of individuals;

- it strengthens the powers of the supervisory authority;
- it sets new rules for the transfer of data outside the European Union;
- it allows the existing registration scheme to be simplified.

The most fundamental differences between the 1984 and 1998 Acts concern the change in the definitions of 'personal data' and 'processing' [289]. The new law is limited to living people and data are only personal if they can be traced back to identifiable persons. The Act does not therefore cover anonymised data. Processing is defined more widely than the 1984 Act to cover any activity from collection to destruction as well as retention. The new Act also applies to the computer processing of any data whether by reference to subject or not. Word processing is also covered more extensively than before. For the first time data protection is extended to personal data held in manual records.

Articles 25 and 26 of the new Act deal with the transfer of personal data across national borders—an area of direct relevance to telemedicine. Provided the transfer meets the other requirements of the Act, it can proceed if the importing country has equivalent data protection measures. This constraint also applies to national amendments to the European Directive so a request for transfer can be refused if the importer does not have similar extensions in place.

After all this legislation, we will conclude Section 6.3 with a more practical look at data security.

6.3.4   Secure Network Access

Telemedicine relies heavily on the transmission of data, video and audio across telecommunication networks, and our discussion demonstrates that secure network access and data transmission are critical to the confidentiality and privacy of personal medical data. Let us deal with network access first.

Clearly, we must assess the consequences (i.e. calculate the risks [290, 291]) of unauthorised access to data to determine the safeguards to put in place. We have to develop a security policy by answering questions such as the following:

- How sensitive are the data we wish to protect?
- What are the consequences of a breach of security?
- Who are the authorised and unauthorised users?
- How vulnerable are the data?
- What are the technical issues?
- Do we wish to eliminate, minimise or simply reduce the threat of unauthorised access?

- How do we balance the needs of authorised users with the constraints imposed by security?

In the UK, these considerations produced an acrimonious debate [292] between the NHS Information Management Group and the British Medical Association concerning access to the dedicated NHS network, the NHSnet [293]. The promise of this network is that patient information will be available electronically to authorised personnel, e.g. doctors, nurses etc., wherever the patient happens to be or the information is needed. The aims of NHSnet security are therefore to facilitate the authorised sharing of data across the network and to prevent unauthorised access and tampering.

The approach adopted to achieve these aims is a Code of Connection [294] which sets out minimum conditions that organisations must meet if they wish to gain access to NHSnet. The basic provisions include:

- access is protected by at least one authentication control (password);
- controls are in place to ensure non-NHS access is available only to authorised users;
- one named individual is made responsible for the security of a connected system;
- all relevant staff are made aware of their responsibilities;
- physical access to NHS-wide termination equipment is controlled;
- all incidents which constitute a threat of security are reported appropriately.

However, the concept of NHSnet was designed before Internet technologies had captured the public imagination and become the *de facto* standard for communication over an intranet [291] (which is essentially what NHSnet is). Hence, the characteristics of NHSnet have had to change to take advantage of the new technologies [295, 296].

The most obvious way of reducing the risk of unauthorised access to computer data across the Internet is to control the traffic across the interface between the NHS local area network and the external Internet. This is the function of a *firewall* [291]. A firewall is a system, or group of systems, that facilitates legitimate traffic across the interface and blocks illegal traffic. Clearly, this task is only possible once an organisation has made a strategic decision as to what access it wants to permit and what it wants to deny. One firewall may favour access while another may block it. One implementation may simply monitor, audit and prioritise access while another may deny all but mission-critical functions such as email.

Generally, firewalls are set up to provide a single point of connection between internal and external networks and configured to prevent unauthenticated and interactive logins from the outside world. It is important to recognise, however, that they cannot protect against traffic that does not go through them, for example, via a modem and dial-up telephone line.

Conceptually, there are two types of firewall. The *network-level firewall* uses a router to make decisions on what to pass or block based on network protocols, typically Internet protocol (IP) addresses. For example, a network-level firewall could be configured to allow all outgoing Internet access from an organisation but to accept incoming web pages only if they come from non-hostile IP addresses.

An *application-level firewall* is more sophisticated and is based on a system comprising a PC with two ports, one for incoming, the other for outgoing, traffic. Appropriate software then analyses traffic on both ports to determine what should pass through the firewall. A typical application is to allow internal users outgoing access to the Internet and incoming access only to the organisation's web pages. The configuration therefore prevents external users from accessing other internal resources.

The advance of NHSnet could have significant implications for the development of telemedicine in the UK. We shall watch these developments with interest.

6.3.5   Secure Data Transmission

A firewall is a means of ensuring that only the right traffic gets through. It does not guarantee that the traffic is itself 'right', i.e. that it has not been intercepted by intruders or eavesdroppers. This intervention, or more strictly the consequences of it, is prevented by message *encryption*. Encryption is therefore a powerful aid to secure telemedicine transactions.

Encryption involves a mathematical algorithm and a key to encode a message so that it is readable only by the transmitter and the receiver. There are two types of encryption algorithm. With *secret key* encryption the sender and the receiver both use the same key to lock and unlock the message. The key is known only to these parties.

In contrast, with *public key* encryption [291, 297] each user has two unique keys, a public key and a private one. You distribute your public key to correspondents and they use this key to encrypt messages they send to you. Messages encrypted with your public key can only be decrypted with your private key so that as long as this key remains secret no one else can read your incoming messages. You can similarly encrypt outgoing messages with your correspondent's public key so that they can decode them with their own private key. Your private key can also be used to encrypt any message you send as a *digital signature* [298]. The recipient can decrypt the signature with your public key to verify your identity and the authenticity of the message.

The power of digital signatures is that they detect even very slight changes to a message. If someone alters a comma to a full stop in the transmitted message (data) or introduces a virus then the signature will no longer verify.

The signature cannot tell you what has changed but it will tell you that the received message is not the same as the transmitted one.

The most common form of public key cryptography is a program by Phil Zimmerman known as *Pretty Good Privacy* (PGP) [297]. PGP is itself based on a public domain algorithm known as RSA after its inventors Rivest, Shamir and Adleman. The US government is not keen on PGP because it allows people to exchange messages that the government cannot decode.

As with all security measures, the value of PGP depends upon secrecy and trust.

The universality of web browsers as interfaces to the Internet and intranets has led to measures to ensure the secure operation of these programs. The most important of these measures is the *Secure Sockets Layer (SSL) Protocol* [291] implemented originally in Netscape's Navigator browser and Commerce Server but now available in other browsers. SSL is a protocol layer between the standard Internet transmission control protocol (TCP/IP) and the application layer protocol, *Hypertext Transmission Protocol* (HTTP). It guarantees secure data communication (server identify, message authentication, encryption and data integrity) from an SSL-enabled server to an SSL-enabled browser. See reference [299] for further details of Internet security.

Secure HTTP (HTTPS) transmissions across the Internet are especially important for commercial transactions. Electronic commerce on the Internet has been a goal ever since the explosion of interest in the Internet in the early 1990s but rival technologies (Mastercard and Visa) delayed market agreement. Eventually, both parties pledged their support for a third protocol called *Secure Hypertext Transfer Protocol* (S-HTTP) developed by Terisa Systems. This agreement brings together the major players in secure transactions and network vendors have blessed the union by ensuring that their switches and routers can handle S-HTTP.

The joint technology, to serve about 700 million customers worldwide, is referred to as *Secure Electronic Transactions* (SET) [299]. SET uses both secret and public key technologies to secure data in transit. It does not provide end-to-end security since it regards the start and finish of transactions as the responsibilities of the buyers and the vendors. For this reason, some experts believe that SET is an incomplete solution to Internet secure transactions.

Developments in secure data transmission over the Internet have profound implications for the future of integrated healthcare in general and telemedicine and telecare in particular.

6.4   ETHICAL AND LEGAL ASPECTS OF THE INTERNET

6.4.1   Patients, Physicians and the Internet

The implications of the Internet have permeated this text, suggesting that it will be a major influence on the way we practise medicine and the way in which patients assume increasing responsibility for their own care. As testimony to its impact, a recent poll [300] has shown that more than 98 million US adults have sought healthcare information online and 75% and those who have access to the Internet use it to find health-related information. This explosive growth brings threats as well as opportunities, and many clinicians are unprepared both technically and mentally for the new patient power and the ethical and legal dilemmas that the new paradigm produces.

For example, physicians now find that they need to provide online services [301] such as web sites, direct email communication, and question/answer sessions to help interpret the information that patients acquire. They are also concerned about the amount of time they need to spend with patients to explain the shear mass of data and the way in which the Internet is reducing the asymmetry of the patient–doctor relationship.

An oft-expressed threat is the uncertain origin and quality of information offered in a frequently anarchic and unregulated environment [302] (see Section 6.4.2). Another perceived threat that remains high on the agenda of concern is the privacy and confidentiality of personal information. Patients (as well as web site developers!) have shown themselves sceptical [303] of claims that information is secure and immune to attack. Patient trust is a key issue and once it is lost it is difficult to recover.

However, the convenience of electronic communication means that despite the many ethical concerns of clinicians, medical advice, email diagnosing [304] and prescribing [305] will become increasingly common, as will the automatic monitoring of conditions and the transmission of test results. While services will be tailored more to individual needs and customised care becomes the norm, the web will also be used to host treatment regimes such as disease management programmes and care protocols, and the depersonalisation of these activities could result in the loss of vital contextual clues and a reduction in the quality of care. A further move in the direction of impersonal care is the tendency of physicians to form groups so that the group is online rather than an individual.

Government must be aware of and respond to these pressures by educating the public and providing a legal framework in which unethical and irresponsible practice can be exposed and the offenders punished. This framework should involve healthcare professionals and industry, and should encourage them to construct ethical codes [306, 307] and act in a self-regulatory manner to minimise malpractice and maximise patient benefits (see Sections 5.2.1 and the rest of Section 6.4).

6.4.2   Ethical Guidelines for Patient Information

Informed users quite naturally expect clinical information on the Internet to be of high quality, i.e. accurate, timely and based on evidence. That is, they expect the content of a web site to be governed by the same principles as scientific and professional publications [303]. Thus, they want to know the names and affiliations of the authors and their declared interests and the date of publication of the web information as well as the names of any sponsors.

Naïve users have less critical faculty and are more easily persuaded of the validity of what they read on a web page. However, all users require information to be presented in ways that facilitate its retrieval so that they can draw the maximum benefit from it. They also need the assurance that any information they themselves provide will remain private and confidential (see Section 6.4.1).

Several organisations have endeavoured to enshrine these principles in guidelines or codes of ethical practice [304, 306, 307] for the construction of Internet web sites. The Hi-Ethics [307] consortium is a voluntary group which aims to:

> unite the most widely used consumer health Internet sites and information providers whose goal is to earn the consumer's trust and confidence in Internet health services.

The objectives of Hi-Ethics are to:

- offer Internet services that reflect high quality and ethical standards;
- provide health information that is trustworthy and up to date;
- keep personal information private and secure, and employ special precautions for any personal health information;
- empower consumers to distinguish online health services that follow these principles from those that do not.

Members agree to adhere to these objectives, to be open in their interactions with consumers and to provide mechanisms for consumer feedback on any relevant issue. They must also recognise and point out the limitations of health web sites and state that these cannot replace the human interaction of a conventional patient–physician relationship.

The intention of Hi-Ethics is to provide Internet users with the consumer protection they deserve while providing content and web site developers with a clear set of rules that can be successfully and accountably implemented.

A similar approach has been adopted by the US clinicians' professional organisation, the American Medical Association. The AMA 'Guidelines for medical and health information sites on the Internet' [306] are intended to remove barriers to the transition towards shared decision making between patient and physician. They cover the same issues as those mentioned above with some additional comments on e-commerce, and they wisely recognise the pace of changing technology by acknowledging that the guidelines will need continuous revision.

6.4.3   Ethics and Legality of Internet Medical Services

To date, the use of the Internet to deliver medical services has been largely restricted to advice in a patient–carer setting [304] or to the dispensing of prescriptions [305]. In the former situation, the value of the online therapy to the patient is clearly dependent on the credentials and expertise of the carer. Even if the qualifications and status of the clinician are above question, (and these may be difficult to assess) it does not follow that this person can exploit the new medium to offer the care that he or she would provide in a traditional consultation. There are also many opportunities for misunderstanding due to the absence of visual clues and the tendency for the mind to fill in knowledge gaps in an idealistic way [304].

These problems point to the need for some sort of accreditation with training and assessment guidelines. King and Poulos [304] address these issues from the standpoint of clinical psychologists and raise concerns about the use of email (therapy) to counsel patients and the need for a better understanding of the medium and its constraints.

Although we have suggested that the impersonal nature of computing and the Internet can raise ethical problems, there are circumstances, particularly in psychiatric and psychological conditions, where the interpolation of a machine between patient and carer can be less threatening to the patient, who may feel less self-conscious and able to exercise greater control over events. These circumstances can be exploited by the skilled practitioner but the skills must be acquired and the education and licensing of qualified therapists must be part of any ethical system using the Internet.

When we turn to prescribing we find that 1 October 2000 is a watershed in the use of the Internet for dispensing drugs. This was the day that the Electronic Signatures in Global and National Commerce Act became law in the USA [305]. While the law does not require private individuals to use or accept electronic signatures as authorisation, it gives such signatures legal enforceability when they are so used.

The 'E-sign' law, as it has become known, requires the presence of an interstate or foreign transaction. Prescribing is clearly a transaction and in modern times the international nature of the pharmaceutical industry almost guarantees the second requirement. Thus, prescriptions signed with electronic signatures are legal documents for the supply of medication just as handwritten prescriptions on paper.

E-sign allows state agencies to specify standards for the accuracy, integrity and access to records but prevents them from substantial regulation of transactions and the reimposition of paper record requirements. E-sign has consequently been regarded by some US states as an assault on their rights and the law has created considerable tension. Furthermore, there is no requirement that the electronic signature bear any relationship to the signer— an 'X' is perfectly acceptable. The law seems certain to make lawyers richer.

6.5   TELEMEDICAL MALPRACTICE

6.5.1   Duty of Care and Clinical Negligence

In most countries with common law jurisdictions, such as the UK, an action for telemedical negligence requires the plaintiff to establish that [308]:

- the defendant (e.g. the teleconsultant) owes him or her a *duty of care* (established via the patient–doctor relationship;
- the duty has been breached, i.e. the teleconsultant was negligent;
- he or she suffered harm (compensatory injury) as a consequence of the negligence.

We will consider each of these conditions in turn since they illustrate well how the law works.

First, the duty of care owed to a telepatient is much the same as that owed to a patient treated by conventional means since it depends upon the nature of the patient–doctor relationship (Section 6.2.2), which is similar in most respects. Thus, the clinician may incur liability at any time after accepting responsibility for the patient's treatment irrespective of any contractual arrangement or payment for care. Where a contract does occur, e.g. in private healthcare, then the conditions of ordinary contract law may also apply although there are few circumstances (possibly equipment unfit for purpose) in which a claim in contract is appropriate.

Beyond these circumstances, there is little case law for telemedicine to define clear precedents. Thus, while the doctor's duty of care is well established, the liability of paramedics, nurses and other non-clinical carers is less certain. Legally, these persons are not expected to have the same level of responsibility as their clinical counterparts [308] but they still owe the patient a duty of care.

The healthcare organisation that employs the doctors and non-clinical carers also owes a duty of care to the patients for whom it provides services. But what is the extent of corporate liability if a UK NHS Trust fails to provide an adequate level of telemedicine or other services because it has financial problems and has to engage in some form of rationing? It has been said that questions of healthcare policy are 'for parliament, not the courts' [308].

This aspect brings us neatly to the second condition—the *standard of care*. The courts have a dual role here: first, to define the appropriate standard of care in any given medical specialism, and second, to determine if the teleconsultant's actions fall short of that standard and constitute negligence.

The test of what constitutes the appropriate standard of care is the Bolam test met in Section 6.2.5, i.e. 'the practice accepted as proper by a responsible body of men skilled in that particular art' [309]. A clinician would not be negligent if he or she departed from accepted practice for good reason, nor if medical opinion was divided on a particular course of treatment. He or she would probably be regarded ·as negligent, however, if there were no valid reasons for departure from established practice and the weight of medical opinion held that the choice or standard of care was deficient and irresponsible.

Interestingly, the Bolam ruling can lead to a switch in the burden of proof in clinical negligence cases. At the outset, the burden may lie with the plaintiff (patient) to establish that the defendant departed from accepted practice. Once this is achieved, the burden of proof then passes to the defendant to justify his or her departure.

Most cases of negligence arise from missed diagnoses since these grounds are easiest to identify (and hindsight is a very exact science!). Examples include not testing a patient for a condition indicated by their history, e.g. failing to check for broken bones in athletes or contraindications in drugs, or mistakes made in prescribing the correct drugs and dosage. These errors are more likely in a teleconsultation because of the remoteness of the patient and the possible involvement of non-clinicians.

Finally, we come to the third condition, the *cause of damage*. It is frequently easier to convince a court that damage has occurred than to prove that the damage was a result of negligence. Thus, if the outcome of a medical condition was likely irrespective of the intervention, e.g. the post-operative death of a patient with life-threatening head injuries, then the courts will find in favour of the defendant. Only if the court is convinced that damage followed directly from the negligence of the defendant, and would not have occurred 'but for' this negligence will the court find for the plaintiff. This is sometimes known as the 'but for' test [308].

6.5.2   Professional Standards and Regulation

The Bolam principle is no arbitrary application of medical opinion swayed by fashion and expediency. Instead, standards of treatment and conduct and advice on good practice are declared by the various professional bodies that regulate the activities of doctors and other healthcare professionals.

In the UK, the General Medical Council (GMC) is the pre-eminent body of this sort [310]. The GMC oversees medical education, maintains a register of doctors, and deals with allegations of professional misconduct and deficient practice. It is a statutory body with considerable powers that are remarkably free from interference by the state or other interested parties. These powers can be traced back to the Medical Act (1858) and to the concordat between the state and doctors as controllers of access to medical care [311].

The process of professional regulation is conducted mainly through the issue of guidelines and the various committees that deal with misconduct (see below). To date, the GMC has issued no guidelines specifically for telemedicine and the advice it gives is based on the practice of conventional medicine.

Prior to 1995, the standard code of practice, *Professional Conduct and Practice: Fitness to Practise* (the Blue Book) [312] placed the emphasis on disciplinary measures. Since then, however, four new booklets under the broad title *Duties of a Doctor: Guidance from the General Medical Council* (see Sections 6.2.2 and 6.2.3 and reference [284]) have taken a more supportive line by disseminating good practice and helping doctors to achieve and maintain appropriate standards.

These booklets cover some areas of particular relevance to teleconsultants. For example, they provide advice to multidisciplinary teams urging them to work constructively with clinical and non-clinical colleagues and reminding them of the crucial constraints on confidentiality. Other advice, referred to earlier (Section 2.3.2) concerns the delegation of responsibilities to non-clinical staff and the need to ensure that they have the competence to discharge their roles.

If situations arise in which good practice and advice are ignored, then the GMC has significant powers to deal with offenders. Cases are heard first by a Preliminary Proceedings Committee which decides on the basis of written evidence and submissions those cases it will refer to the Professional Conduct Committee. Only 5% of the cases heard by the Preliminary Committee are referred on, the Committee either sending doctors a warning or taking no further action. Those cases that are referred comprise allegations that fall into three categories [310]:

- criminal conviction for a non-trivial offence;
- practice that is seriously deficient (e.g. negligence);
- serious professional misconduct.

There is a right of appeal from the Professional Conduct Committee to the Privy Council but the latter will rarely interfere.

Stanberry [310] discusses these and other issues of standards and regulations in far greater depth and erudition than we do here and we happily refer you to his book for more detail.

6.5.3   The Law Applicable to Telemedical Equipment

Stanberry's expertise extends also to the legal aspects of telemedical equipment and its fitness for purpose [313]. He charts a sure path through the intricacies of UK and European legislation but it is not one we shall follow far. A few tentative steps are all we shall take.

Surprisingly, as late as 1994 in the UK, the safety of medical devices was the responsibility of the Department of Health (DoH) operating a voluntary scheme of manufacturer registration combined with the reporting by the NHS of 'adverse incidents'. These arrangements are gradually being replaced by a unified system of European Directives embodied in UK law. The bedrock of this legislative framework is the Consumer Protection Act (1987) dealing with general liability for manufactured products. This Act has been followed by three Directives targeted at medical devices:

- The Active Implantable Medical Devices Regulations, which came into force on 1 January 1993. These regulations apply mainly to powered implants such as pacemakers.
- The Medical Devices Regulations Directive came into full force on 13 June 1998 and covers most other devices from bandages to hip prostheses.
- The *In-vitro* Diagnostic Medical Devices Directive was adopted in 1997 and covers any device, reagent, kit (e.g. pregnancy testing) or instrument for the examination of human body substances.

The second sanction on Medical Devices Regulations is clearly the most relevant to telemedicine although the others can apply to equipment recommended during teleconsultations. The Regulations apply to CT scanners, X-ray, ultrasound etc. although not to videoconferencing equipment used in non-telemedical applications. In the fullness of time, all such devices (including new videoconferencing and related equipment) must display the 'CE' mark showing that they conform to appropriate standards of safety, quality and performance. Conformity to these standards depends upon a manufacturer's own quality assurance systems, and a series of international standards known as EN 46000 defines quality procedures (including sterilisation) for the production of medical devices. This series is implemented together with the more widely applicable ISO 9000 standards and manufacturers accredited to these standards enjoy considerable protection against actions for negligence.

Since 1994, inspection to ensure adherence to these standards has been the responsibility of the newly formed *Medical Devices Agency* (MDA). The MDA is also responsible for manufacturer registration and incident reporting, as previously discharged by the DoH, as well as for the general implementation and promotion of the European Directives (see reference [313] for details). In addition, the MDA advises the DoH, commissions evaluations and publishes hazard bulletins.

The MDA has identified the repeated causes of adverse incidents with medical devices as:

- poor quality, obsolete or worn-out devices;
- incompatibility with ancillary equipment;
- poor documentation;
- inappropriate use;
- inadequate training;
- mistakes in servicing or lack of servicing.

To minimise these risks, the MDA advises manufacturers and service providers to ensure that devices are suitable for their intended purpose, properly understood by professional users, and maintained in a safe and reliable condition. By law, these organisations must report to the MDA any incidents covered by these causes that could seriously injure a patient's health. The MDA also encourages a more proactive role in reporting less serious incidents to establish good practice and avoid repeated problems.

So where does the liability for negligence due to equipment failure or malfunction in a teleconsultation lie? The basic principle of product liability in English law is that a plaintiff has a cause for action if an injury or loss occurs as a consequence of defective products. The liability may arise from a contractual obligation or from a duty of care. The defendant can be the equipment manufacturer, a service supplier using the equipment, an assembler for poor workmanship, or a repairer not exercising due care.

A wise precaution for a manufacturer is to discharge his obligation to provide equipment fit for purpose by warning his customers that they should arrange for the equipment to be tested before it is put into routine use. Similarly, in the absence of such a warning, a service provider, assembler or repairer would be well advised to carry out such testing to assure themselves that the equipment functions properly in normal operating conditions. If sued by a telepatient, any one of these parties could then claim that they had taken all reasonable precautions.

If, however, a plaintiff (telepatient) is injured after he or she had chosen to ignore a warning of potential danger then it is unlikely that any action for negligence brought against a defendant would succeed. Similarly, if a service provider misused a telemedicine system, then he or she could not easily pass responsibility for ensuing damage to the manufacturer. Finally, failure to discharge their supervisory duties adequately might also lay the MDA open to an action for negligence.

These comments apply mainly to operational equipment failure or malfunction but what if the fault lies in equipment design or construction? Surely these faults are the responsibility of the manufacturer? Well, yes and no—this is the law after all! The courts like to refer to 'development defects' by which they mean defects that were impossible to foresee at the time the equipment was designed. The equipment may actually have been manufactured to this same design at a much later date in which case it may still be subject to development defects.

It is difficult to sustain an action against a defendant for such defects although it is incumbent on a manufacturer to revise a design in line with the latest technical (and medical) thinking, or issue an appropriate warning about restricted usage. This continuing duty of care also implies that manufacturers should recall equipment that is clearly unsafe (due to faulty design or any other factor) and they would be liable to prosecution if they failed to do so.

6.5.4   Operational Risks Due to Technology

In Chapter 5 of his book, Stanberry [308] gives a good account of what he refers to as the clinical risks to telemedical malpractice. These operational risks are precisely those identified by the MDA as the main causes of adverse incidents (Section 6.5.3). Analysis of these causes shows that they fall into two categories: inadequacies due to technology and those due to personnel insufficiencies. We shall treat these causes under the separate category headings, technology in this section, and personnel in the next.

We can distinguish four main technology risks:

- quality of images;
- lack of suitable equipment;
- malfunctioning equipment;
- inadequate guidelines.

Quality of Images

A patient has the right to expect that a consultant can draw the same, correct conclusions from an image on a telemedicine display screen as he or she can decide from a conventional face-to-face consultation. This is especially important for pathology, dermatology and radiography investigations. As we saw in Chapter 3, considerable work has been done by radiologists to define the degree of data compression that can be tolerated before X-ray image quality suffers to the point of producing unacceptable clinical errors. Other disciplines need to follow this lead to assess and manage the risks of error and litigation.

Lack of Suitable Equipment

The responsibility for providing the equipment for a healthcare service lies with the appropriate health services managers. In the UK, this is an unenviable accountability given the constraints on the NHS and, as pointed out in Section 6.5.1, courts are largely sympathetic to the plight of managers in these circumstances. This sympathy would almost certainly evaporate, however, if an external report on the service provision had recommended that a health authority or Trust should increase the amount and range of telemedical equipment and it had not complied with the directive. A similar legal fate might befall an organisation that had failed to improve its management of a telemedicine facility, leading to injury of a patient.

Malfunctioning Equipment

The breakdown of computer or video equipment is unfortunately one of the more common features of telemedicine. The faults are usually simple and traced to the interfaces between the various components. However, the effects can be just as devastating and as fatal as more serious defects (see also Section 6.5.3).

Inadequate Guidelines

A guideline can be viewed as a bridge between the technology and the participants in the teleconsultation. We explored the role of clinical process guidelines in Section 2.3.2 and the more managerial practice guidelines in Section 5.4.7. We refer you back to these sections for the necessary detail. Both types of guideline are used to establish a high-quality and consistent standard for the telemedical consultation. The guidelines determine the process of teleconsultation and the documentation provides a record of therapy, prescriptions, drug dosages, future plans etc. This combination of protocol and record of action provides a powerful audit trail that can be of considerable value in any legal dispute. The protocol might also be of benefit to the patient's case if it was not followed correctly but the advantages of a protocol to a defendant invariably outweigh the risks.

6.5.5   Operational Risks Due to Personnel

We can distinguish five main risks to telemedical practice arising from deficiencies in the care team, some of which we have touched upon in earlier chapters (2 and 4):

- poor communication;
- limited ability;
- poor training;
- improper delegation;
- unclear responsibility.

Poor Communication

A protocol is helpful in identifying the stages of a teleconsultation where special care is needed to ensure clarity of communication between participants. Deaf and elderly patients are particularly prone to misunderstandings, as are patients (and doctors) whose native tongue is not the language of the consultation. Even if everyone speaks the same language then accent, dialects, and distorted audio and video images can conspire to introduce misconceptions, with potentially serious implications. Reviewing the record of a teleconsultation (see above) is also helpful to check for errors, for example, in prescriptions and drug doses, directions to the patient and follow-up appointments. There should also be a protocol for reporting errors that do occur since an audit of mistakes is valuable in preventing further occurrences and establishing good practice. Naturally, this requirement presumes a culture in which the reporting of errors is not discouraged by fears of speculative litigation.

Limited Ability

The employment of under-qualified (and unqualified) practitioners in clinical radiology reflects the shortage of posts in this area [314]. This is a worrying situation since, as one study [315] showed, non-specialist doctors had an error rate in detecting potentially significant abnormalities that was nearly 40% higher than consultant radiologists. Hopefully, teleradiology and greater access to consultants will begin to alleviate such problems. Even so, the problem is symptomatic of a health service under stress due to underfunding and/or poor management.

Poor Training

The training of teleconsultants has been mentioned many times throughout the book (see Chapter 5 in particular). Ideally, training should include not only the clinical aspects of telemedical treatment [316] but also the ability to use the technology effectively [217] as well as interpersonal and interviewing skills. Failure to address these issues can lead to accusations and court proceedings for negligence.

Improper Delegation

The delegation of care to less well-qualified subordinates and the necessity of establishing their competence has also come to our attention several times throughout our discussion. If a task is beyond the competence of a delegate then the ultimate responsibility reverts to the delegating clinician. If the delegate is competent to discharge the task then he or she shoulders the responsibility. Either way, it is essential for the patient's safety and well-being that subordinates make it clear if they are proficient in the tasks they are asked to perform. As we have seen, telemedicine may unwittingly increase the opportunities for improper delegation, and therefore litigation, due to the remote nature of the care process.

Unclear Responsibility

The requirement of clear responsibility for a telepatient's care is no different from that of a patient treated by conventional medicine. An issue for tele-medical care may be the number of medical staff involved in the process, and due diligence on the part of the lead clinician is necessary to ensure that each member of the (often frequently changing) team is aware of their own responsibilities and those of other members. The patient should also know who is in charge of his or her care. These are simple precautions to avoid malpractice or negligence complaints.

6.6 JURISDICTIONAL ISSUES

6.6.1 State Regulation of Telemedicine

The majority of the legal issues we have considered so far tend to fall into two well-defined categories: those issues that have a common basis with conventional medicine, and those that are specific to telemedicine (usually as a consequence of the remote nature of the care process) [280]. There is, however, a third category that we must now consider for which the legal implications depend upon the local laws and practice of medicine. States (a general term covering federal as well as sovereign states) may differ widely in the requirements they impose upon clinicians and the penalties they exact for malpractice or other contraventions of the law. These conflicts are referred to as *jurisdictional issues* [317].

The archetypal example of this geographical conflict is the United States of America, where the disunited and uncoordinated laws of over 50 states make jurisdictional issues a major barrier to the progress of telemedicine (Section 2.5). The central issue is the licensure of clinicians (Section 6.6.2) who can practise telemedicine but the implications are many.

For example, a claim for negligence can only be filed if a patient–doctor relationship has been established since only then can a duty of care be breached. Most states would agree that a duty of care arises once a patient agrees to treatment and the clinician agrees to provide it, whether the clinician receives reimbursement or not. However, is it less clear if such a relationship is established through an emergency hotline or via an Internet discussion group [318].

Again, if a telepatient in one state seeks redress for negligence against a teleconsultant from another state then where should the claim be filed? Should justice be sought in the patient's state, in the clinician's state or somewhere else (e.g. a Federal court) [267]? In the USA, the diversity of legislation has led to 'forum shopping', i.e. the filing of a claim in a court with the most 'pro-plaintiff' laws or injunctions sought by defendants to ensure trials take place in courts with the most 'pro-doctor' laws.

In the USA, the federal (Second) Restatement of Conflict of Laws states [267]:

> In an action for personal injury, the local law of the state where the injury occurred determines the rights and liabilities of the parties, unless, with respect to the particular issue, some other state has a more significant relationship.

The 'unless' obviously allows for 'conflicting' interpretations.

In English law a dispute about jurisdiction produces a stay of proceedings and the case is moved to a forum where the interests of the parties and the ends of justice are better served [317]. This forum will usually be the one with the most substantial link with the case but other considerations apply,[4] e.g.:

- availability of witnesses;
- convenience;
- expense;
- residence of the parties.

When telemedicine takes place across national borders then there are likely to be even more opportunities for legal discord [319]. Which laws apply, those of the country in which the telepatient is harmed, or those of the country where the teleconsultant practises medicine? What if the teleconsultant is licensed to practice in one country but gives emergency advice from another?

Potentially, even more problematical are jurisdictional decisions regarding telemedical malpractice at sea. The usual view is that the forum of jurisdiction is that of the country whose flag a merchant ship is flying. This decision may be modified if a ship is sailing through, or anchored within, the territorial waters of another nation, in which case that nation may be able to claim jurisdiction.

Stanberry [317], because of his special expertise in maritime law, raises other variations on this seafaring theme and the interested reader can cruise the pages of his book.

Evidently, although there are common approaches to cross-border (state and international) telemedicine law the current situation tends towards the chaotic. The G8 group of nations has tried to address this problem and has instituted the G8-ENABLE Project [320] which has sought to identify and overcome the barriers to health within a global information society. The group's 1998 report proposes a *Memorandum of Understanding* to establish a code of *Telemedicine Good Practice* that attempts to harmonise laws concerning security and confidentiality, standards of care, remuneration, intellectual property rights etc. There is a long way to go yet.

6.6.2   Licensure and Accreditation

To practise medicine it is widely held that a person must have received the relevant education and training and reached a pre-set standard. Eventually, he or she is given a licence to practise. However, there is no universal agreement about either the length or content of training, or the standards needed to

---

[4]   The seemingly endless dispute over the venue for the trial of the alleged terrorists who caused the crash of the Pan-American jet over Lockerbie in Scotland is an example of the legal wrangling that can ensue as the litigants seek justice or advantage for their claims.

qualify as a doctor. Thus, physicians accept that to practise in a country other than the one they originally qualified in they will usually need to take additional examinations, e.g. the United States Medical Licensing Examination (USMLE), and satisfy other bureaucratic requirements such as providing evidence of their primary qualifications and the standards achieved. The process may require the clinician to appear before a country's licensing board and take examinations in that country—a potentially time-consuming and expensive business.

It is more difficult to accept that similar precautions are needed to practise medicine in different states of the same federal country but that is precisely the situation in the USA. State Medical Practices Acts require anyone who wishes to practise medicine in a state to have a practice licence from that state [317]. Some states will grant a licence against passing scores in the National Board of Medical Examiners examination or the Federation Licensure examination [321] while others, e.g. California, demand an oral examination.

Telemedicine has raised awareness of the issues underscoring this mismatch of legislation [322]. Is the licensure issue [323]:

- a regulatory barrier to telemedicine or a basic patient safeguard against incompetent or impaired practitioners;
- a restriction on commerce and trade or an essential requirement that allows states to protect the health, safety, and welfare of its individuals;
- a basic standard of medical practice or an attempt to preserve physicians' traditional patterns of referral;
- another case of the federal government overreaching or the yielding of another patchwork quilt of state laws and regulations?

Endeavours to steer a course between these opposing views have only added to the confusion. Thus, some states (e.g. Illinois, Utah) have created exemptions for out-of-state physicians who assist in emergencies. Others (e.g. Oklahoma and Indiana) extend this exception to 'irregular or infrequent' teleconsultations [324].

While many of these laws are not restricted to telemedicine, some states have passed specific telemedicine legislation, e.g. Florida restricts teleconsultations involving unlicensed out-of-state clinicians to those based on electronic images, and Arizona requires written and verbal patient consent for the participation of out-of-state doctors. One state, Kansas, demands that out-of-state teleconsultants have a Kansas medical licence and other states are looking at similar provisions. This situation is a nightmare for teleconsultants since the unwary could easily find themselves practising without a licence ('practising bare') and without insurance.

With such confusion, there is a clear need for interstate licensure based on mutual recognition. This is the same principle that allows doctors to practise in any member countries of the European Union or the states of Australia [324, 325]. Interstate licensure based on common requirements in education, training, certification and other conditions may be difficult to achieve, however. An alternative based on a compact of mutual recognition with individual states retaining their power over educational and competency requirements may be easier to agree.

The long-term goal must surely be a federal licensure system, perhaps restricted to telemedicine. All states now oblige doctors to graduate from an approved medical school and pass the USMLE qualification so that educational requirements are fairly standard. In 1996, the Federation of State Medical Boards proposed a Model Act [322, 324] that would allow an out-of-state clinician to obtain a state licence to treat telepatients 'regularly or frequently' across state lines. The licence would not allow the doctor to practise medicine from within the state unless he or she held a full and unrestricted licence. No states have yet adopted the Model Act and indeed the American Medical Association at its House of Delegates meeting in June 1996 called for full licensure in each state, leading to the flurry of activity noted above.

The outcome of these deliberations is difficult to foresee. One thing is sure, however: financial and anti-federal factors will vie for importance with ethical and patient-centred considerations.

Licensure can be regarded as a passport for suitably qualified persons to enter and practise a profession. *Accreditation*, *credentialing* or *certification* is the granting of a licence that recognises more advanced knowledge and competencies. Accreditation status can be awarded to persons or to organisations who can then undertake certain types of work or offer specified services that have been approved by an external body. By inspection or some other form of examination the accrediting body guarantees that the persons and/or the services achieve pre-set levels of quality. The accrediting body may be a government organisation, e.g. the Medical Devices Agency, a professional institute, e.g. the Royal College of Surgeons, or a commercial company, e.g. Microsoft.

Telemedicine is probably not sufficiently well-defined as a discipline to justify professional accreditation as a 'telemedicine specialist' at the present time. However, the commercial advantage and professional kudos of a quality mark have led organisations to seek some form of accreditation and also to require specialists to perform a minimum number of teleconsultations a year to retain their professional status [280].

6.6.3   Clinician Reimbursement

We will end this section on the jurisdictional issues with a very quick look at physician reimbursement.

In the USA, physicians are reimbursed for the medical services they provide directly by patients, or indirectly by managed care organisations under insurance arrangements, or from the government's Medicare and Medicaid schemes. The schedule of what is allowable and what is not under the indirect schemes is therefore of considerable interest to doctors.

The established practice before telemedicine arrived on the scene was to reimburse doctors only for face-to-face consultations. That is now changing. Teleradiology is reimbursed nationally (Section 1.3.2) and Medicaid reimbursement for telemedical consultations is provided in Arkansas, Georgia, Montana and West Virginia. Non-videoconferencing applications such as remote cardiac and foetal monitoring, telepathology and teleradiology have been nationally reimbursed by Medicare, for some time [4]. From January 1999, Medicare reimbursement is also available for telemedicine services in rural counties (Section 5.2.2 and reference [215]).

As noted, the US General Accounting Office found no evidence to support the Health Care Financing Administration's assertion that offering fee-for-service reimbursement of telemedicine services to Medicare patients would vastly increase expenditure in the USA [214]. Others [326] have questioned whether reimbursement is the big issue that it is made out to be, and further relaxation to allow controlled reimbursements seems likely.

6.7 INTELLECTUAL PROPERTY RIGHTS

The term *intellectual property rights* (IPR) is a generic term covering the commercial value and goodwill associated with inventions, computer software, trade marks and designs as well as literary, aesthetic and artistic works [327]. IPR law attempts to steer a course between encouraging innovation and protecting the authors of the ensuing designs and products from unscrupulous exploitation by others. There is always a danger that protection can create monopolies and stifle further innovation so that there is an ongoing tension between these two motives.

This tension leads to some complex and often confusing and conflicting legislation and case law, much of it with limited relevance (at the present time) to telemedicine equipment and software. We shall therefore confine ourselves to a discussion of patents and licensing and copyright law. Most of our discussion applies to the UK. Readers needing more expertise and details on IPR law and its relationship to telemedicine should consult Stanberry's book [328], which is a valuable source of material and references.

6.7.1 Patent Law

Following the UK Patents Act (1977), patents on products or processes can be applied for in several ways, depending on whether the patent is required to be British, European or international in scope. Scientific theories and mathematical techniques are held to be in the public domain and therefore not patentable (but note the dispute on attempts to patent gene technology inventions). Inventions against public interest are also outside the scope of the Act, as are literary, aesthetic and artistic works since these fall under the control of copyright law (Section 6.7.2).

Outside of these restrictions, a patentable item must satisfy the following key conditions;

- *Novelty*: the equipment is regarded as a new invention if its design has not previously been published or used.
- *Inventive step*: an invention must involve a design element which is not obvious to those familiar with the concepts. The step may have been published or used before but not patented.
- *Industrial application*: an invention must be capable of industrial application (hence excluding aesthetic items).

If the authors of the patent meet the necessary conditions then they are granted a 20-year monopoly to exploit the patent. During this time no other person or organisation may legally copy or otherwise take advantage of the patented design or applications without the express permission of the authors. The Patent Act also sets out the actions that will infringe a patent if carried out without this permission. A patent is infringed [328]:

- where the invention is a product, another person makes, disposes of, offers to dispose of, uses or imports the product or keeps it whether for disposal or otherwise;
- where the invention is a process, another person uses the process or he offers it for use in the United Kingdom when he knows, or it is obvious to a reasonable person in the circumstances, that its use there without the consent of the proprietor would be an infringement of the patent;
- where the invention is a process, another person disposes of, offers to dispose of, uses or imports any product obtained directly by means of that process or keeps any such product whether for disposal or otherwise.

The word 'dispose' in these rather arcane paragraphs is not meant in the conventional usage of 'throw away' but in the more general sense of the proverb, 'man proposes, God disposes' to cover any eventuality that might constitute infringement.

It should be noted, however, that an action otherwise regarded by these statements as an infringement is not so if it is a 'one-off' event, an experiment, or done privately and for non-commercial purposes [328].

Those who infringe patents through ignorance are usually brought to see the error of their ways before cases come to court. Others who blatantly ignore patents for profitable gain clearly place themselves outside the law and are usually dealt with expeditiously. It is the third group of infringers, those who studiously try to modify patented designs and products to avoid the penalties of the Patent Act, who offer considerable scope for conflict in the interpretation of its provisions.

The scope for infringement is reduced considerably by providing a carefully constructed specification of the equipment in the patent application. Drawing up a specification is a skilled task particularly since there are stringent limitations on amending a patent. The rationale of the patent claim must spell out clearly the way in which the claim meets the key conditions noted above. Thus, the claim for a new device would emphasise novelty whereas an improvement of an existing device would stress how inventiveness is achieved.

The industrial application is particularly important since it should cover all likely applications of the equipment. For example, someone seeking a patent on a videoconferencing system customised for telemedicine (if such a patent were possible) should include non-telemedicine applications where the design and manufacture are essential for the ancillary uses. Otherwise a competitor could claim that the patent did not extend to a new application.

A manufacturer wishing to exploit some competitor's creative ideas should also remember that the combination of features defining a product is as important as the individual characteristics. Thus, the new manufacturer will infringe the patent if he or she simply adds new features to the full set of existing ones even if the revision produces a better product. To avoid infringement, the new product must leave out or replace one or more features of the patented product. Stanberry [328] quotes several cases, including the famous *Epilady* case, which illustrate this point well.

6.7.2   Patents and Licensing

One legal way for a manufacturer to benefit from someone else's skills and creativity is to obtain a licence to manufacture and/or market the patented equipment. The exclusive licence is the most attractive form of licence to the licensee, but not necessarily to the licensor. This type of licence gives the licensee the right in law to prevent any person (including the licensor) from selling the patented product within the licensee's territory. It also prevents the licensor from granting licences for that product to any other persons operating within the same territory.

The benefits of an exclusive licence to the licensor are that he can put his full marketing and manufacturing support behind a single licensee and avoid the hassle of dealing with multiple contractors. The exclusivity of the licence may also mean the licensee works harder to make the relationship a success. However, the benefits are generally greater for the licensee since he has effectively got the owner of the patent to eliminate much of his competition. The price of the licence or the royalty fees should reflect this benefit.

The most serious risk to the patent owner is the danger of granting too wide a territorial advantage to the possessor of an exclusive licence. For example, a licensor granting an exclusive worldwide licence to a licensee effectively prevents himself from selling his product directly anywhere outside of his own country—not good business sense unless the licence has a restricted timescale. Both parties to the licence should also appreciate the potentially monopolistic nature of such a contract, which may contravene anti-competition and freedom of movement of goods laws.

Stanberry [328] gives an interesting discussion of the matters that licensor and licensees should consider to protect their individual interests when devising a licence. These include:

- *Non-disclosure agreements*: to ensure confidentiality of the licensor's expertise and 'know-how' before, during and even perhaps after the termination of the licence;
- *Duration of licence*: so that the licence can be renegotiated by both parties to reflect their circumstances in changing market conditions.
- *Patent enhancements*: the licensee will wish to take advantage of any new patents and associated upgrades produced by the licensor, and the latter will wish to have a 'grant-back' clause in the licence agreement giving him access to innovations introduced by the licensee.
- *Related intellectual property*: the licensee might wish to have access to the licensor's other registered or unregistered designs, or to their trade mark, brand name or 'look-and-feel' if the products are well known.

6.7.3 Copyright Law

The purpose of copyright law is to protect literary, aesthetic and artistic works by granting their authors and publishers periods of legal protection during which other persons may not reproduce these works without their permission. Within the European Union the protection period lasts for the lifetime of the author (or the longest living author in a joint work) plus 70 years. Authors, or their successors, can sue anyone abusing their copyright.

Unlike patents, copyright confers no monopoly of use status. Neither is there any formal registration process as with patents. Instead, the onus is on the author to prove ownership.

The relevance of copyright law to telemedicine is that in the UK computer programs and databases are classified as literary works[5] so that intellectual property rights can be extended to these forms. Various Acts have confirmed this protection, the current legislation arising from the Copyright, Design and Patents Act (1988) amended by the European Software Directive to produce the Copyright (Computer Programs) Regulations (1992).

Copyright rests with the author(s) of a program or with their employer unless a contract between the parties states otherwise. The copyright holder has the exclusive right to reproduce, load, run, transmit or store the program,

---

[5] Not all countries regard computer programs as literary works. Some require the work to involve the reader directly and for the work to be more inspirational than code to operate a machine before it is afforded the protection of copyright [328].

in part or in whole. The same protection extends to subsequent versions of the program provided the modified forms contain substantial parts of the original. This ownership remains with the author throughout the lifetime of the program, which is why when you 'purchase' a program you are buying only a licence to use it and not acquiring ownership or the accompanying copyright.

As described, the situation seems to be a straightforward application of the laws of property. The difficulties arise when there is dispute over the interpretation of the word 'substantial'. How much underlying code needs to be modified before the program is essentially a new one and not covered by the original copyright? Suppose the code of two programs performing similar tasks is dramatically different but the user interfaces and their look-and-feel are very similar? What if the code of a program is translated line by line into a different programming language?

The European Software Directive states that [see reference 328]:

> Ideas and principles which underlie any element of a computer program, including those which underlie its interfaces, are not protected.

This statement demonstrates that copyright applies only to the expression of an idea and not to the idea itself. Put another way, copyright is not concerned with originality of thought but with the originality of the expression of thought. Thus, copying the plot of a play would not of itself infringe copyright but if all the characters and scenes were identical to the original then that most certainly would.

Extrapolating this concept to computer programs implies that copying the overall structure of a program does not violate copyright but copying it line for line does.[6] If this seems reasonable then suffice to say that courts, especially in the USA, have found otherwise and case law is at best inconsistent. Courts will always look at the intention of the defendant in a copyright claim. If the intention is simply to disguise exploitation of the plaintiff's original work then the plaintiff's action is likely to succeed (*cf* patent licences, Section 6.6.2).

The concept of originality comes up again in a rather different way when considering the copyright protection of factual compilations such as databases [328, 329]. These compilations are increasingly important to healthcare and telemedicine as information technology and information management play ever-increasing roles.

---

[6]   The classical dispute between Apple Computers and Microsoft Corporation in the USA over the 'Windows' interface illustrates the difficulties faced by courts. Apple tried to assert copyright over its windows metaphor interface running on its own hardware, claiming that Microsoft had breached that copyright by transporting the concepts to Intel-based hardware. The action might have succeeded except that after a long battle the court took the view that the windows interface was so ubiquitous that it was essentially in the public domain and users expected software to conform to this *de facto* standard. Similar disputes may attend the advent of the Internet.

The US Copyright Act [329] defines a compilation as:

A work formed by the collection and assembling of pre-existing materials or of data that are selected, coordinated, or arranged in such a way that the resulting work as a whole constitutes an original work of authorship.

The European Software Directive has an essentially similar definition [328] but the US alternative has the merit that its includes the all-important term 'original'. This term was crucial to a recent judgement in the US Supreme Court when a telephone company unsuccessfully defended its alleged right of copyright over the white pages of its telephone directory. The court did not feel that the compilation had sufficient originality to classify as a literary work.

The creative aspect of database construction that confers copyright is the judgement exercised to select or reject the database entries. The protection applies to the database rather than to its contents (*cf* medical records, Section 6.2.4) and lasts for 15 years from the completion of the database. There is no real indication as to how the UK or European courts will respond to the provisions of the Directive in this context.

6.8 SUMMARY

In Chapter 6 we have seen that:

- The guiding principle behind the legal perspective of confidentiality is the concept that information is held to be confidential if its release has the potential to injure a person either emotionally or materially. This concept applies whether or not a contract or other formal relationship exists between the confider and the confidant.
- The duty of confidence lies at the heart of the patient–doctor relationship. Patients who reveal personal information to their doctors must be able to trust them not to divulge the same information to others incidental to the care process.
- When patients give consent to disclosure of information about themselves, doctors must make sure that patients understand what will be disclosed, and the reasons and circumstances for disclosure.
- Doctors must also make sure that patients are informed whenever information about them is likely to be disclosed and they must normally respect requests by patients to withhold information. Disclosure should be restricted to information essential for the purpose, and health workers should understand that information is given to them in confidence.
- Current thinking on medical records tends towards a division of ownership in which the healthcare organisation 'owns' the physical form of the record and the patient 'owns' the information contained within.

- Every competent adult has a right to refuse or consent to available medical treatment or healthcare. Clinicians in charge of care must obtain a patient's consent before proceeding with the treatment. The point at which consent is given is difficult to judge.
- The protection and security of medical data in the UK are covered by the Data Protection Act (1984), the Computer Misuse Act (1990) and the Data Protection Act (1998).
- Secure network access is provided by an appropriate code of connection and the use of firewalls. The NHSnet is the national healthcare intranet in the UK.
- Secure data transmission is achieved by encryption, digital signatures, and over Internet protocols by secure sockets layer and secure electronic transactions technology. Pretty Good Privacy is a popular method of public key encryption.
- An action for telemedical negligence requires the plaintiff to establish that the defendant owes him or her a duty of care, the duty has been breached, and he or she suffers harm as a consequence of the negligence.
- The Bolam test determines the appropriate standard of care.
- The General Medical Council is the relevant UK professional body for regulating standards of care via advice on good practice and disciplinary measures for non-adherence.
- The law relating to the suitability of telemedical equipment in the UK is administered by the Medical Devices Agency (MDA). The MDA is responsible for manufacturer registration and incident reporting, and it advises the Department of Health, commissions evaluations and publishes hazard bulletins.
- Operational risks due to technology in teleconsultations include quality of images, lack of suitable equipment, malfunctioning equipment and inadequate guidelines.
- Operational risks due to personnel in teleconsultations include poor communication, limited ability, poor training, improper delegation and unclear responsibility.
- In the United States of America the disunited and uncoordinated laws of over 50 states make jurisdictional issues a major barrier to the progress of telemedicine. The central issue is the licensure of clinicians who can practise telemedicine but the implications are many.
- Licensure, the licence to practise medicine in a state, is confused by the ability of telemedicine to facilitate healthcare across state, federal and international boundaries.
- The reimbursement of clinicians for advice and treatment rendered across state boundaries is a source of friction and concern but the issues may not be as important as they seem.
- Patent law in the UK demands that a patentable product or process is novel, contains an inventive step, and has an industrial application. Scope

for patent infringement is reduced by a carefully drawn specification covering the design and uses of the item.

- Patent licensing allows a manufacturer to benefit from someone else's skills and creativity. An exclusive licence to market or manufacture a patented item is of considerable benefit to the licensee.
- The purpose of copyright law is to protect literary, aesthetic and artistic works by granting their authors and publishers periods of legal protection against reproduction of these works without permission. Within the UK, computer programs and databases are classified as literary works.

TELEMEDICINE BOOKS AND WEB SITES

BOOKS

This selection of recent books is confined to texts that deal specifically with telemedicine and telehealth applications. Many references to these subjects also appear in more general texts on health and medical informatics.

Bashshur R, Sanders J L and Shannon G W, *Telemedicine, Theory and Practice*, Thomas, Springfield, IL, 1997

This book covers a wide range of aspects including the context of telemedicine, the technology, clinical applications, telemedicine systems and future developments.

Coiera E, *Guide to Medical Informatics, the Internet and Telemedia*, Hodder and Stoughton, London, 1997

Coiera's book is concerned with the broad range of information and communication technologies in healthcare and the general area of health informatics. Topics include the role of information in clinical practice, the Internet, the Cochrane Collaboration, evidence-based protocols, data mining and knowledge discovery so that the book contains much that is relevant but peripheral to telemedicine.

Darkins A W and Cary M A, *Telemedicine and Telehealth: Principles, Policies, Performance, and Pitfalls*, Springer, London, 2000

The authors explore how the medical, social, cultural and economic dimensions associated with emerging digital data networks will affect future healthcare services. The book offers a framework for healthcare professionals to develop networks and solutions in telemedicine and telehealth.

Bauer J C and Ringel M A, *Telemedicine and the Reinvention of Healthcare*, McGraw-Hill, New York, 1999

A book from the Executive Management series; this text aims to bring managers and the general public up to speed on current trends in e-health.

Geyman J P, Norris T E and Hart L G, *Textbook of Rural Medicine*, McGraw-Hill, New York, 2001

The title indicates that the book covers more than telemedicine and telehealth but there are several chapters of relevance. An overview defines the roles of rural patient, physician and care team as well as indicating the basis of links to public health and health policy. A chapter on the organisation and management of rural healthcare covers telemedical issues.

Field M J (ed), *Telemedicine: A Guide to Assessing Telecommunications for Health Care*, Committee on Evaluating Clinical Applications of Telemedicine, Institute of Medicine, Washington, DC, 1996

A comprehensive text covering similar ground to the present book. The authors define terms, trace the development of telemedicine, and consider the technology. The book is strong on the strategic and evaluation aspects of telemedicine and has good sections on licensure and remuneration.

Goldstein D E, *E-Healthcare: Harness the Power of Internet, E-Commerce and E-Care*, Aspen, Gaithersburg, MO, 2000

Goldstein introduces the e-healthcare revolution in the context of the new e-commerce business model. The chapters discuss the diverse audience, available services, legal aspects and trends of modern electronic (telemedical) healthcare.

Howard G S, *Introduction to Internet Security*, Prima Publishing, Roseville, CA, 1995

This is one of a whole glut of books on the technical aspects of Internet security but this one is relatively undemanding. The contents include privacy versus freedom of information, the fundamentals of computer security, security on the Internet, WAN and LAN security and encryption etc. The book is easy to read and a good pointer to weightier tomes.

Hart T and Fazzini L, *Intellectual Property Law*, Macmillan, Basingstoke, 1997

Although not concerned with telemedicine, this is a useful, inexpensive book that details the essentials of patent law and copyright in a readable way. It also covers trademarks in greater depth than we do within the present book and is very up to date and authoritative.

Healy J, *Medical Negligence*, Sweet and Maxwell, London, 1999

Most books on this subject are a few short of 1000 pages and cost a fortune. At 200 pages and a little over £20, Healy's book is an exception. It explores the area of medical negligence, concentrating on claims under common law. It makes useful international comparisons with jurisdictions in the UK and other English-speaking countries.

Nicholson L (ed), *The Internet and Healthcare*, 2nd edn, Health Administration Press, Chicago, IL, 1999

This book outlines the capabilities of Internet technology in healthcare, discussing security and other implementation concerns. This second edition contains two new chapters on physician integration and call centres.

Slack W, *Cybermedicine: How Computing Empowers Doctors and Patients for Better Health Care*, Jossey Bass, San Francisco, CA, 1997

This book takes a broad view of telemedicine by concentrating on how patients and physicians can make use of online resources for better healthcare. As a consequence, the author is able to make out a credible case for the computer as a humanising influence in healthcare.

Stanberry B A, *The Legal and Ethical Aspects of Telemedicine*, Royal Society of Medicine, London, 1998

This text has been a constant companion throughout the writing of this book, particularly the latter chapters. It has a good account of the origins and development of telemedicine but its strength, as the title suggests, is the medico-legal aspects of the subject; licensure and intellectual property rights are particularly well handled. There is a strong emphasis on UK and European legislation together with seafaring law but it is really the only text that does justice to the legal issues raised by telemedicine. Thoroughly recommended.

Wootton R and Craig J (eds), *Introduction to Telemedicine*, Royal Society of Medicine, London, 1999

Professor Richard Wootton is the acknowledged expert of UK telemedicine with great experience in the area. The various authors consider the background to telemedicine, the main applications, the success factors (a very strong section), benefits and limitations, and the future. The book has a uniform, practical approach and is particularly useful for anyone contemplating setting up a telemedicine service. It has a chapter by Ben Stanberry on the medico-legal aspects which serves as a useful introduction to his own book. This is another timely source that will stand the test of time.

INTERNET RESOURCES

Arent Fox

Arent, Fox, Kintner, Plotkin and Kahn is a US law firm specialising in health law, particularly e-health and telemedicine. The resource is very comprehensive, covering Federal and state legislation as well as practitioner views on all legal and other aspects of telemedicine. The web site has recently been updated and reorganised. The strongly hierarchical structure means that the articles you now want may be embedded at low levels with lengthy URLs. It is an excellent service, though. The URL is http://www.arentfox.com.

Department of Defense Telemedicine

This is the US site of the high-spending military services in the USA. There is a list of projects, a newsletter, a calendar of events, and links to other military sites and publications. Recent developments have resulted in the setting up of a Telemedicine and Advanced Technology Research Center (TATRC) with a web site at http://www.tatrc.org/.

Federal Telemedicine Gateway

The US Federal Gateway is a source of information about federal programmes in telemedicine. As well as the ubiquitous links to other sources, including non-federal ones, there is information on funding and other advice to the would-be telemedicine researcher. The URL is http://www.cbloch.com.

Telemedicine Information Exchange (TIE)

TIE is the foremost web site for telemedicine. It is based at Oregon Health Science University in the USA and supported by the National Library of Medicine. The site has a bibliographic database of over 7000 articles, information on over 150 telemedicine programmes, the dates of international meetings, data on telemedicine vendors and much, much more. This is *the* place to start to find out about telemedicine. The URL is http://tie.telemed.org.

UK Telemedicine Information Service

This web site contains a comprehensive list of past and present UK projects in telemedicine and telecare. It is based at the University of Portsmouth. There is a bulletin board for the exchange of comments and links to other sites along with a few documents. The URL is http://www.tis.bl.uk/.

The European Health Telematics Observatory

This web site is a compendium of material and links to a vast range of telemedicine activities within Europe, many of which are funded by the European Union. Some of the links are to national affiliated sites. There is an emphasis on leading edge technology and standards and the site is always up to date, with current issues and pointers to the future. Legal issues are also covered. The URL is http://www.ehto.be.

REFERENCES

1. Telemedicine Research Centre, *What is Telemedicine?*, Oregon Health Sciences University, Portland, OR, 1999. See also the web page at http://tie.telemed.org/ WhatIsTelemedicine.asp
2. Perednia D A and Allen A, Telemedicine technology and clinical applications, *Journal of the American Medical Association*, **273** (6), 483–488, 1995
3. American Telemedicine Association, *Telemedicine: A Brief Overview*, Congressional Telehealth Briefing, Washington, DC, 1999. See also the web page at http:// www.atmeda.org/news/overview.html
4. Mitchell J, *Fragmentation to Integration: National Scoping Study for the Telemedicine Industry in Australia*, Department of Industry, Science and Tourism, Canberra, ACT, 1998. This report can be downloaded from the web site http:// www.noie.gov.au/publications/1988.htm
5. Nagendran S, Moores D, Spooner R and Triscott J, Is telemedicine a subset of medical informatics?, *Journal of Telemedicine and Telecare*, **6** (Suppl 2), 50–51, 2000
6. Mitchell J, *From Telehealth to E-Health: The Unstoppable Rise of E-Health*, Department of Communications, Information, Technology and the Arts, Canberra, 1999. This report can be downloaded from the web site at http://www.noie.gov.au/ projects/ecommerce/ehealth/rise_of_ehealth/unstoppable_rise.htm
7. Goldstein D E (ed), *E-Healthcare: Harness the Power of Internet, E-Commerce and E-Care*, Aspen, Gaithersburg, MO, 2000
8. Nicholson L (ed), *The Internet and Healthcare*, 2nd edn, Health Administration Press, Chicago, IL, 1999
9. CEC DG XIII, *Research and Technology Development on Telematics Systems in Health Care*, AIM 1993, Annual Technical Report on RTD, Health Care Brussels, 1993
10. Wootton R and Craig J (eds), *Introduction to Telemedicine*, Royal Society of Medicine, London, 1999, Chapter 1
11. Stanberry B A, *The Legal and Ethical Aspects of Telemedicine*, Royal Society of Medicine, London, 1998, Chapter 1
12. Benschoter R, CCTV-pioneering Nebraska medical centre, *Educational Broadcasting*, October, 1–3, 1971
13. Bashshur R L, *Technology Serves the People; the Story of a Cooperative Telemedicine Project by NASA, the Indian Health Service and the Papago People*, US Government Printing Office, Washington, DC, 1980
14. Jutras A, Teleroentgen diagnosis by means of videotape recording, *American Journal of Roentgenology*, **82**, 1099–1102, 1959
15. Murphy R L Jr and Bird K T, Telediagnosis: a new community health resource;

observations on the feasibility of telediagnosis based on 1000 patient transactions, *American Journal of Public Health*, **64** (2), 113–119, 1974

16. Foote D R, Satellite communication for rural health care in Alaska, *Journal of Communication*, **27** (4), 173–182, 1977

17. House A M, and Roberts J M, Telemedicine in Canada, *Canadian Medical Association Journal*, **117** (4), 386–388, 1977

18. Watson D S, Telemedicine, *Medical Journal of Australia*, **151** (2), 62–66, 68, 71, 1989

19. Grigsby J and Kaehny M M, *Analysis of Expansion to Care through Use of Telemedicine and Mobile Health Services. Report 1; Literature Review and Analytic Framework*, Centre for Health Policy Research, Denver, CO, 1993

20. Allen A and Grigsby J, Fifth annual programme survey, part 2: Consultation activity in 35 specialties, *Telemedicine Today*, **6** (5), 18–19, 1998

21. Falconer J, Telemedicine systems and telecommunications, in Wootton R and Craig J (eds) *Introduction to Telemedicine*, Royal Society of Medicine, London, 199, Chapter 2

22. Randall N, *The Soul of the Internet*, Thomson, Boston, MA, 1997, Chapter 8

23. Iseman C J, Broadband options open wireless worlds for telemedicine, *Telemedicine and Telehealth Networks*, **4** (1), 41–42, 1998

24. Coyle D, *The Weightless World*, Capstone, Oxford, 1997

25. Tapscott D, *The Digital Economy*, McGraw-Hill, New York, 1996

26. Brecht R M, Gray C L, Peterson C and Youngblood B, The University of Texas Medical Branch—Texas Department of Criminal Justice telemedicine project: findings from the first year of operation, *Telemedicine Journal*, **2** (1), 25–35, 1996

27. Stanberry B A, *The Legal and Ethical Aspects of Telemedicine*, Royal Society of Medicine, London, Chapter

28. News item, Telemedicine defence medical services, *Computer Bulletin*, January, 24, 1999

29. Berry F C, Telemedicine and the army, *Army Magazine*, April, 1996

30. Editorial, *Time Magazine*, **52** (2), 20, 1998

31. News item, Home health care via telemedicine, *Telemedicine Today*, **3** (3), 18–19, 31, 1995. See also the web version at http://telemedtoday.com/articlearchive/articles/homehealthcare.htm

32. Mitchell J, *Best Practice in Telemedicine: An Evaluation of The Queen Elizabeth Hospital Renal Dialysis Telemedicine Project 1995–1996*, John Mitchell and Associates, Adelaide, 1996. See also the version of the article at the web site at http://www.jma.com.au/tqehrep2.htm

33. Mitchell J G, Disney A P S and Roberts M, Renal telemedicine to the home, *Journal of Telemedicine and Telecare*, **6**, 59–62, 2000

34. Johnson J, Managed care in the 1990s: providers' new role for innovative health delivery, *Hospitals*, **66**, 26–30, 20 March 1992

35. Allen A and Stein S, Cost effectiveness of telemedicine, *Telemedicine Today*, **6**, 10–12, 14–15, 1998. See also the web version at http://telemedtoday.com/articlearchive/articles/cost_effectiveness_of_telemedici.htm

36. Department of Health, *The New NHS: Modern, Dependable*, Cm 3807, HMSO, London, 1997. See the web site at http://www.official-documents.co.uk/document/doh/newnhs/contents.htm

37. NHS Executive, *Information for Health*, Department of Health Publications, Wetherby, 1998. See the web site at http://www.doh.gov.uk/nhsexipu/strategy/index.htm

38. Ariff I and Chuan G C, *Multimedia Super Corridor*, Leeds, Kuala Lumpur, 1998

39. Ministry of Health, *Malaysia's Telemedicine Blueprint*, Government of Malaysia,

Kuala Lumpur, 1997. This document and many other links of interest related to the Multimedia Super Corridor (MSC) Programme can be found at the web site http://www.mdc.com.my/msc/flagship/tm.html

40. See the UK Telemedicine Information Service web site at http://www.tis.bl.uk
41. See the European Health Telematics Observatory home page at http://www.ehto.org
42. Wachter G and Grigsby B, External vs internal funding: does it matter who pays the bills?, *Telemedicine Today*, **5** (1), 30–32, 1997
43. Pedersen S, Telemedicine in the future, in Wootton R and Craig J (eds), *Introduction to Telemedicine*, Royal Society of Medicine, London, 1999, Chapter 13
44. American Telemedicine Association, *The Global Application of Video Conferencing in Health Care: Executive Summary*. See the web page at http://www.atmeda.org/news/globalexe.html
45. Tachakra S and Haig A, How to do a telemedical consultation, in Wootton R and Craig J (eds), *Introduction to Telemedicine*, Royal Society of Medicine, London, 1999
46. Hurwitz B, Clinical guidelines: proliferation and medicolegal significance, *Quality in Health Care*, **3**, 37–44, 1994
47. Freeman K, Wynn-Jones J, Groves-Phillips S and Lewis L, Teleconsulting: a practical account of pitfalls, problems and promise. Experience from the TEAM project group, *Journal of Telemedicine and Telecare*, **2** (Suppl 1), 1–3, 1996
48. Mitchell J, *From Telehealth to E-Health: The Unstoppable Rise of E-Health*, Department of Communications, Information Technology and the Arts, Canberra, 1999, p 11. See also Mitchell J and Disney A P S, Clinical applications of renal telemedicine, *Journal of Telemedicine and Telecare*, **3**, 158–162, 1997
49. Mitchell J, *From Telehealth to E-Health: The Unstoppable Rise of E-Health*, Department of Communications, Information Technology and the Arts, Canberra, 1999, p 32
50. Mitchell J, *From Telehealth to E-Health: The Unstoppable Rise of E-Health*, Department of Communications, Information Technology and the Arts, Canberra, 1999, p 32. See also the web site at http://www.medeserv.com.au/index.cfm
51. Mitchell J, *From Telehealth to E-Health: The Unstoppable Rise of E-Health*, Department of Communications, Information Technology and the Arts, Canberra, 1999, p 19. See also the web site at http://www.cme.net.au
52. See the National Electronic Library of Health web site at http://www.nelh.nhs.uk
53. See the National Library of Medicine web site at http://www.nlm.nih.gov
54. See the Cochrane web site at http://www.cochrane.de
55. Young H L, Tele-education, in Wootton R and Craig J (eds), *Introduction to Telemedicine*, Royal Society of Medicine, London, 1999, Chapter 5
56. Young H L, Satellite-delivered medical education and training for Central Europe: A TEMPUS project, *Journal of Telemedicine and Telecare*, **2**, 14–19, 1996
57. Hasman A and Albert A, Education and training in health informatics: guidelines for European curricula, *International Journal of Medical Informatics*, **45** (1–2), 1997, 91–110
58. Mantas, J (ed), *Health Telematics Education, State of the Art Report on Education and Telematics in the Health Care Sector*, Studies in Health Technology and Informatics, vol 41, IOS Press, Amsterdam, 1997, pp 3–7
59. Rao M, *Internet is an Emerging Key Component of Telemedicine Infrastructure in Developing Nations*, see web site at http://oneworld.org/news/reports99/telemedicine.htm

60. See, for example, the Dorset Health Authority web site at http://www.dorset. swest.nhs.uk/index.htm

61. Mitchell J, *From Telehealth to E-Health: The Unstoppable Rise of E-Health*, Department of Communications, Information Technology and the Arts, Canberra, 1999, pp 14–15

62. See Vera Bradover's web site for lymphoma sufferers at http://www.geocities.com/ ~vera_b/index.html and the Cancer Research Campaign's CancerHelp UK site on a wider range of conditions at http://www.cancerhelp.org.uk

63. Lewis L, Roach R B and Haynes E, A low-cost approach to public health education using multimedia packages, *Journal of Telemedicine and Telecare*, **6** (Suppl 2), 41–43, 2000

64. Fahrenberg J and Myrtek M, *Ambulatory Assessment*, Hogrefe and Huber, Göttingen, 1996

65. Friedman R H, Kazis L E, Jette A *et al*, A telecommunications system for monitoring and counselling patients with hypertension, *American Journal of Hypertension*, **9**, 285–292, 1996

66. Ahring K, Joyce C, Ahring N and Farid N, Telephone modem access improves diabetes control in those with insulin-requiring diabetes, *Diabetes Care*, **15**, 971–975, 1992

67. Shanit D, Cheng A and Greenbaum R A, Telecardiology supporting the decision making process in general practice, *Journal of Telemedicine and Telecare*, **2**, 7–13, 1996

68. Casey F, Brown D, Craig B G, Rogers J and Mulholland H C, Diagnosis of neonatal congenital heart disease by remote consultation using a low-cost telemedicine link, *Journal of Telemedicine and Telecare*, **2**, 165–169, 1996

69. Allen A, Bowersox J and Jones G G, Current state of telesurgery, *Telemedicine Today*, June 1997. See also the version at http://www.telemedtoday.com/ articlearchive/articles/telesurgery.htm

70. Demartines N, Freiermuth O and Mutter D, Knowledge and acceptance of telemedicine in surgery: a survey, *Journal of Telemedicine and Telecare*, **6**, 125–131, 2000

71. Tachakra S, Mullett S T H, Freij R and Sivakumar A, Confidentiality and ethics in telemedicine, *Journal of Telemedicine and Telecare*, **2**, 68–71, 1996

72. Standing Committee of European Doctors (CP), *Ethical Guidelines in Telemedicine*, April 1997. See the web site at http://www.utu.fi/research/mircit/ ethics.html

73. Hjelm M, Benefits and drawbacks of telemedicine, in Wootton R and Craig J (eds) *Introduction to Telemedicine*, Royal Society of Medicine, London, 1999, Chapter 10

74. General Medical Council, *Professional Conduct and Discipline: Fitness to Practice*, GMC, London, 1993

75. Johnson S (ed), *Pathways of Care*, Blackwell, Oxford, 1997

76. Norris A C, Care pathways and the new NHS, *Journal of Integrated Care*, **2**, 78–83, 1998

77. Bridge, G E and Norris, A C, *Care Pathways and their Relationship with UK Healthcare Strategy*, European Healthcare Management Association Conference, Dublin, June 1998

78. Benger J, Protocols for minor injuries telemedicine, *Journal of Telemedicine and Telecare*, **5**, 26–45, 1999

79. Randles T J, *Telemedicine's Impact on the Medical Diagnostic Process*, PhD Thesis, Georgia State University, 1997

80. Richards T, Partnership with patients, *British Medical Journal*, **316**, 85–86, 1998

81.   Elford D R, Telemedicine in northern Norway, *Journal of Telemedicine and Telecare*, **3**, 1–22, 1997

82.   Mitchell J, *Fragmentation to Integration: National Scoping Study for the Telemedicine Industry in Australia*, Department of Industry, Science and Tourism, Canberra, ACT, 1998. See Chapter 4 for the USA, Chapter 5 for South-east Asia, and Chapter 6 for Australia

83.   American Telemedicine Association, *The Global Application of Video Conferencing in Health Care, Section 2: Medical Applications and Benefits*. See also the web page at http://www.atmeda.org/news/globalsec2.htm

84.   See for example the Cyberhospital web site at http://www.cyber-hospital.org.uk

85.   Baldwin G, Attention shoppers, *American Medical News*, 19 April 1999. See also the web site at http://www.ama-assn.org/sci-pubs/amnews/pick_99/tech0419.htm

86.   Johnston B, Wheeler L and Deuser J, Kaiser Permanente Medical Centre's pilot tele-home health project, *Telemedicine Today*, **5** (4), 16–19, 1997

87.   Wheeler T, Corrections-based telemedicine programs top most-active list, *Telemedicine Today*, **6** (3), 40, 41, 44, 1998

88.   Collins B and Sypher H, Developing better relationships in telemedicine practice: organizational and interpersonal factors, *Telemedicine Today*, **4** (2), 27, 42, 1996. See also the version at http://www.telemedtoday.com/articlearchive/articles/developingbetterrelations.htm

89.   Yellowless P, How not to develop telemedicine systems, *Telemedicine Today*, **5** (3), 6–7, 17, 1997. See also the web version at http://telemedtoday.com/articlearchive/articles/hownottodeveloptelemedicine.htm

90.   Yellowless P, Successful development of telemedicine systems—seven core principles, *Journal of Telemedicine and Telecare*, **3**, 215–222, 1997

91.   Yellowless P, How to be successful at telemedicine, in Wootton R and Craig J (eds) *Introduction to Telemedicine*, Royal Society of Medicine, London, 1999, Chapter 7

92.   Western Governors' Association Telemedicine Action Report, 1994 and 1998. See the web site at http://www.westgov.org/wga/publicat/combar4.htm

93.   The Telemedicine Information Exchange (TIE) is based at Oregon Health Science University and supported by the National Library of Medicine. The web site is at http://tie.telemed.org

94.   Brown N, Information on telemedicine, in Wooton R and Craig J (eds) *Introduction to Telemedicine*, Royal Society of Medicine, London, 1999, Chapter 12

95.   Tanriverdi H and Iacona C S, Diffusion of telemedicine: a knowledge barrier perspective, *Telemedicine Journal*, **5** (3), 223–244, 1999

96.   See the University of Montana, Network Montana Project web site at http://www.nmp.umt.edu/technical/recommendations/video%20conferencing.htm

97.   Sisk J E and Sanders J H, A proposed framework for economic evaluation of telemedicine, *Telemedicine Journal*, **4**, 31–37, 1998

98.   Crowe B L, Cost-effectiveness analysis of telemedicine, *Journal of Telemedicine and Telecare*, **4** (Suppl 1), 215–222, 1998

99.   Mori S, Nishida H and Yamada H, *Optical Character Recognition*, Wiley, New York, 1999. See also the useful survey of OCR from a librarian's viewpoint by Haigh S, *Optical Character Recognition (OCR) as a Digitization Technology*, at the web site http://www.nlc-bnc.ca/publications/1/p1-23be.html

100.   Kientzle T, *A Programmer's Guide to Sound*, Wiley, New York, 1998

101.   See the excellent PC Technology Guide article on computer sound at the web site http://www.pctechguide.com/11sound.htm

102.   See the excellent PC Technology Guide article on scanners at the web site http://www.pctechguide.com/18scanners.htm

103. See the excellent PC Technology Guide article on digital cameras at the web site http://www.pctechguide.com/19digcam.htm

104. Ruggiero C, Teleradiology: a review, *Journal of Telemedicine and Telecare*, **4** (Suppl 1), 25–35, 1998. See also Ruggerio C, *A Teleradiology Primer*, at the web site http://www.telemedtoday.com/articlearchive/articles/ateleradiologyprimer.htm

105. Tachakra S, Colour perception in telemedicine, *Journal of Telemedicine and Telecare*, **5**, 211–219, 1999

106. See the Columbia Audio and Video Technology web site at http://www.cs.columbia.edu/~hgs/rtp/glossary.htm   v

107. Wang J and Naghdy G, Three novel lossless image compression schemes for medical image archiving and telemedicine, *Telemedicine Journal*, **6**, 251–260, 2000

108. Della Mea V, Pre-recorded telemedicine, in Wootton R and Craig J (eds) *Introduction to Telemedicine*, Royal Society of Medicine, London, 1999, Chapter 3

109. See the paper by TeamSolutions, *Video Conferencing Standards and Terminology*, at the web site http://www.teamsolutions.co.uk/tsstds.html

110. See the paper by Agans D, *A Primer on Video Conferencing Standards*, Fletcher Allen, 1997 at the web site http://www.vtmednet.org/telemedicine/stand.htm

111. Ash A, Telemedicine: technology and equipment enabling new models of healthcare delivery, *Informatics in Healthcare Australia*, **6** (3), 90–96, 1997

112. Phillips V L, Temkin A J, Vesmarovich S H and Burns R, A feasibility study of video-based home care for clients with spinal cord injuries, *Journal of Telemedicine and Telecare*, **4**, 219–223, 1998

113. Rosen E, *The History of Desktop Telemedicine*, at the web site http://www.telemedtoday.com/articlearchive/articles/historydesktoptm.htm

114. See the PictureTel home page at http://www.picturetel.com

115. See the paper by TeamSolutions, *Desktop Video Conferencing*, at the web site http://www.teamsolutions.co.uk/video.html

116. Blignault I, Multipoint videoconferencing in health: a review of three years' experience in Queensland, Australia, *Telemedicine Journal*, **6**, 269–274, 2000

117. Young J W R, *Displays in Picture Archiving and Communication Systems*, 1998. See the web page at http://www.agfamedical.com/publications/ucsf98/displays.asp

118. Krupinski E, LeSuer B, Ellsworth *et al*, Diagnostic accuracy and image quality using a digital camera for teledermatology, *Telemedicine Journal*, **5**, 257–263, 1999

119. Loane M A, Gore H E, Corbett R *et al*, Effect of camera performance on diagnostic accuracy, *Journal of Telemedicine and Telecare*, **3**, 83–88, 1997

120. Bondmass M, Bolger N, Castro G and Rogers L O, The effect of home monitoring and telemanagement on blood pressure control among African Americans, *Telemedicine Journal*, **6**, 15–23, 2000

121. Brebner J A, Ruddick-Bracken H and Brebner E M, The diagnostic acceptability of low bandwidth transmission for tele-ultrasound, *Journal of Telemedicine and Telecare*, **6**, 335–338, 2000

122. Lamminen H, Mobile satellite systems, *Journal of Telemedicine and Telecare*, **5**, 71–83, 1999

123. National Technology Transfer Centre, *High Data Rate Satellite Communications to Reach Rural and Distant Areas*. See the web page at http://www.nttc.edu/telmed/scfact.html

124. Altrudi R, Gandsas A, Montgomery K and Miglianini G, In-flight monitoring of vital signs by Internet, *Prensa Medica Argentina*, **85** (1), 76, 1998. See also the web page at http://www.mednets.com/teleproducts.htm

125. Kincade K, Wireless hits the ground running, *Telemedicine and Telehealth Networks*, **5** (6), 14–18, 1999
126. Held G, *Data Over Wireless Networks*, Osborne/McGraw-Hill, Berkeley, CA, 2000
127. See the WAP tutorial published on the Internet by the International Engineering Consortium (IEC) at http://www.iec.org/tutorials/wap/
128. Bates A, *The Wireless Web in Healthcare*, InPharm.com, 2000. See the version at http://www.inpharm.com/knowhow/estrategy/webmark_019.html
129. Monson H, *Bluetooth Technology and Implications*, SysOpt.com, 1999. See the version of this article at http://sysopt.earthweb.com/articles/bluetooth/index.html
130. Buckingham S, *An Introduction to the General Packet Radio Service*. See article at web site http://www.gsmworld.com/technology/yes2gprs.html
131. See the abstract of the article, *Mobile Telecoms Update, 2H April 2000*, IDC, Framingham at http://www.marketresearch.com/product/display.asp?ProductID=271155
132. Ibe O C, *Essentials of ATM Networks and Services*, Addison-Wesley, Reading, MA, 1997
133. Dhawain G, *Enabling Remote Access*, McGraw-Hill, New York, 1998
134. Orpanoudakis S C, Kaldoudi E and Tsiknakis M, Towards a digital radiology department—technological advances and clinical evaluations, *European Journal of Radiology*, **22**, 205–217, 1996.
135. Grey P, *Open Systems*, McGraw-Hill, Maidenhead, 1991
136. Reed T, Dam it! How to harness EMR power, *Healthcare Informatics*, April, 51–53, 1997. See also http://www.healthcare-informatics.com/issues/1997/04_97/dam.htm
137. See papers in a special issue of the *British Journal of Healthcare Computing and Information Management*, **14** (1), 1997
138. Bernard C A, Benda R, Mercando A D *et al*, Effectiveness of the fax electrocardiogram, *American Journal of Cardiology*, **7**, 294–295, 1994
139. Loula P, Rauhala E, Erkinjutti M *et al*, Distributed clinical neurophysiology, *Journal of Telemedicine and Telecare*, **3**, 89–95, 1997
140. Halliday B E, Bhattacharyya A K, Graham A R *et al*, Diagnostic accuracy of an international static imaging telepathology consulting service, *Human Pathology*, **28**, 17–21, 1997
141. Owens D R, Telemedicine in screening and monitoring of diabetic eye disease, *Journal of Telemedicine and Telecare*, **3** (Suppl 1), 89–90, 1997
142. Nordrum I, Telepathology: is there a future?, *Telemedicine Today*, **4** (2), 24–26, 1996
143. Wootton R, Real-time telemedicine, in Wooton R and Craig J (eds) *Introduction to Telemedicine*, Royal Society of Medicine, London, 1999, Chapter 4
144. Freedman S B, Direct transmission of electrocardiograms to mobile phone for management of a patient with acute myocardial infarction, *Journal of Telemedicine and Telecare*, **5**, 67–79, 1999
145. Ricke J, Kleinholz L, Hosten N *et al*, Telemedicine in rural areas: experiences with medical desktop conferencing via satellite, *Journal of Telemedicine and Telecare*, **1**, 224–228, 1995
146. Engum B, Nordum I, Ericcson H *et al*, Remote frozen section service. A pathology project in northern Norway, *Human Pathology*, **22**, 514–518, 1991
147. Reponen J, Ilkko E, Jyrkinen L *et al*, Digital wireless radiology consultations with a portable computer, *Journal of Telemedicine and Telecare*, **4**, 201–205, 1998
148. Baer L, Elford R and Cukor P, Telepsychiatry at forty: what have we learned?, *Harvard Review of Psychiatry*, **7**, 7–17, 1997

149. Buist A, Coman G, Silvas A and Burrows G, An evaluation of the telepsychiatry service in Victoria, Australia, *Journal of Telemedicine and Telecare*, **6**, 216–221, 2000

150. Brennan J A, Kealy J A, Gerardi L H *et al*, Telemedicine in the emergency department: a randomized control trial, *Journal of Telemedicine and Telecare*, **5**, 18–20, 1999

151. Beecham L, First NHS walk-in health centres announced for England, *British Medical Journal*, **319**, 214, 1999. See also the web page at http://www.bmj.com/cgi/content/full/319/7204/214/d

152. Lavery R F, Allegra J R, Cody R P *et al*, A prospective evaluation of glucose reagent test strips in the pre-hospital setting, *American Journal of Emergency Medicine*, **9**, 304–308, 1991

153. Darkins A, Dearden C H, Locke L G *et al*, An evaluation of telemedical support for a minor treatment centre, *Journal of Telemedicine and Telecare*, **2**, 93–99, 1996

154. Beach M, Goodall I and Miller P, Evaluating telemedicine for minor injuries units, *Journal of Telemedicine and Telecare*, **6** (Suppl 1), 90–92, 2000

155. Branger P, van't Hooft A and van der Wouden H C, Coordinating shared care using electronic data interchange, *Medinfo*, **8** (Part 2), 1660, 1995

156. Harno K, Paavola T, Carlson C and Viikinkoski P, Patient referral by telemedicine: effectiveness and cost analysis of an intranet system, *Journal of Telemedicine and Telecare*, **6**, 320–329, 2000

157. Torok M, Turi Z and Kovacs F, Ten years clinical experience with telemedicine in prenatal care in Hungary, *Journal of Telemedicine and Telecare*, **5** (Suppl 1), 14–17, 1999

158. Doolittle G C and Allen A *et al*, Practising oncology via telemedicine, *Journal of Telemedicine and Telecare*, **3**, 63–70, 1997

159. Stern J, Heneghan C, Sclafani A P *et al*, Telemedicine applications in otorhinolaryngology, *Journal of Telemedicine and Telecare*, **4** (Suppl 1), 74–75, 1998

160. Mitchell J, *Rural Telemedicine to the Home: An Evaluation of The Queen Elizabeth Hospital Renal Telemedicine Network 1997–1998*, John Mitchell and Associates, Adelaide, 1998

161. Pettersen H, Reorganization of diagnostic imaging in south Sweden: realization and cost-effectiveness, *Academic Radiology*, **5** (Suppl 2), S315–316, 1998

162. Hyer R N, Telemedical experiences at an Antarctic station, *Journal of Telemedicine and Telecare*, **5** (Suppl 1), 87–89, 1999

163. McLaren P M and Ball C J, Interpersonal communications and telemedicine: hypotheses and methods, *Journal of Telemedicine and Telecare*, **3** (Suppl 1), 5–6, 1997

164. Henderson I, Vanlohuizen K and Fenske T, Remote cardiac rehabilitation, *Journal of Telemedicine and Telecare*, **6** (Suppl 2), 28–30, 2000

165. See the background to the Telematics Applications programme web site at: http://www.acad.bg/ftp/Cordis/telematics_2c/tele_tide/tide_workplan/A0128ENH.HTM

166. Gott M, *Telematics for Health*, Radcliffe Medical Press, Oxford, 1995

167. Spurr L and Begg J, *Hand-held Technology for Hands-on Clinicians*, Proceedings of the Second APAMI/Fifth HIC97 Conference on Health and Medical Informatics, Sydney, August, 1997

168. Warner I, Introduction to telehealth home care, *Home Healthcare Nurse*, **14**, 791–796, 1996

169. Mahmud K and Lenz J, The personal telemedicine system, a new tool for the delivery of healthcare, *Journal of Telemedicine and Telecare*, **1**, 173–177, 1995

170. Sixsmith A J, An evaluation of an intelligent home monitoring system, *Journal of Telemedicine and Telecare*, **6**, 63–72, 2000

171. Tang P and Venables T, 'Smart' homes and telecare for independent living, *Journal of Telemedicine and Telecare*, **6**, 8–14, 2000

172. Celler B, Earnshaw W and Ilser E, *Remote Monitoring of Health Status of the Elderly at Home, Preliminary Results of a Five Month Trial*, in Proceedings of Fifth National Health Informatics Conference, Sydney, 1997

173. DeConno F and Martini C, Video communication and palliative care at home, *European Journal of Palliative Care*, **4**, 174–177, 1997

174. Doolittle G C, A cost measurement study for a home-based telehospice service, *Journal of Telemedicine and Telecare*, **6** (Suppl 1), 193–195, 2000

175. Allen A, Doolittle G, Boysen C D *et al*, An analysis of the suitability of home health visits for telemedicine, *Journal of Telemedicine and Telecare*, **5** (2), 90–96, 1999

176. Balas E A and Iakovidis I, Distance technologies for patient monitoring, *British Medical Journal*, **319**, 1309–1311, 1999

177. Crouch R and Dale J, Telephone triage identifying the demand (part 1), *Nursing Standard*, **12** (34), 33–38, 1998

178. Locher M E, Ambulance telemedicine, *News Channel 9*, 13 January 2000. See the web page at http://www.newschannel9.com/vnews//947740304

179. Harrison D I, Draugalis J R, Slack M K *et al*, Cost-effectiveness of regional poison control centres, *Archives of Internal Medicine*, **156**, 2601–2608, 1996

180. Clark T, *Drugstores Want Crackdown on Rogue Sites*, CNET. See the article at the web site at http://news.cnet.com/news/0-1007-200-340582.html

181. Angaran D M, Telemedicine and telepharmacy: current status and future implications, *American Journal of Health-system Pharmacy*, **56** (14), 1405–1426, 1999. See also the version at the web site http://ashp.org/public/pubs/ajhp/vol56/num14/telemedicine.html

182. Royce R, *Managed Care*, Radcliffe Medical Press, Oxford, 1997

183. Royce R, *Managed Care*, Radcliffe Medical Press, Oxford, 1997, Chapter 2

184. Dakins D R, Market targets: 1997, *Telemedicine and Telehealth Networks*, **3** (3), 25–29, 1997

185. Leighty J, Midwest health system invests in telemedicine to cure managed care ills, *Telemedicine and Telehealth Networks*, **21** (11), 11, 13, 1996

186. Davies P, Kansas Blue Cross payment policy yields home healthcare savings, *Telemedicine and Telehealth Networks*, **3** (4), 12–14, 1997

187. Hunter D J and Fairfield G, Disease management, *British Medical Journal*, **315**, 50–53, 1997

188. Richards T, Disease management in Europe, *British Medical Journal*, **317**, 426–427, 1998

189. Craig J, Loane M and Wootton R, Disease management and health outcomes, *Disease Management and Health Outcomes*, **6**, 121–130, 1999

190. Dalton M T, *Managed Care Environment*, PhD Thesis, Walden University, 1996

191. See the NIVEMES home page and update web site at http://www.atkosoft.com/nivemes.htm and http://www.ehto.org/ehto/journal/issue5/nivemes.html

192. Bagshaw M, Telemedicine in British Airways, *Journal of Telemedicine and Telecare*, **2** (Suppl 1), 36, 1996

193. McDonald A, Sky is the limit in a shrinking world, *European Hospital Management Journal*, **3** (1), 66–68, 1996

194. See the article, *Biomedical Sensors and Telemetry for Remote Monitoring of Patients*, at the web site http://www.nttc.edu/telmed/bmfact.html

195. Gates W and Hemmingway C, *Business@The Speed of Thought*, Warner, New

York, 1999, Chapter 21. See also the extensive web site including information on telemedicine at http://www.speed-of-thought.com/getting/explore_airforce.html

196. Vassallo D J, Buxton R N, Kilbey J H and Trasler M, The first telemedicine link for the British Forces, *Journal of the Royal Army Medical Corps*, **144**, 125–130, 1998

197. Caputo M P, *The Applications of Digital Satellite Communications in Conducting Telemedicine*, MS Thesis, University of Houston, TX, 1994

198. Garshnek V, Logan J S, and Hassell L H, *The Telemedicine Frontier: Going the Extra Mile*, 1998. See the web page at http://www.quasar.org/21698/knowledge/telemedicine_frontier.html

199. Garshnek V and Burke F M Jr, Applications of telemedicine and telecommunications to disaster medicine: historical and future perspectives, *Journal of American Medical Informatics Association*, **6** (1), 26–37, 1999

200. Fisk M (ed), *Alarm Systems and Elderly People*, The Planning Exchange, Glasgow, 1989

201. Thornton P and Mountain G, *A Positive Response: Developing Community Alarm Services for Older People*, Joseph Rowntree Foundation, York, 1992

202. Brownsell J, Bradley D A, Bragg R, *et al*, Do community alarm users want telecare?, *Journal of Telemedicine and Telecare*, **6**, 199–204, 2000

203. Press Release, *Telehealth and Telemedicine will Henceforth be Part of the Strategy for Health for All*, World Health Organization, 23 December 1997, Geneva. See also the WHO web site at http://www.who.int and the web page at http://www.who.int/archives/inf-pr-1997/en/pr97-98.html

204. Fujimoto M, Miyazaki K and Von Tunzelmann N, Complex systems in technology and policy: telemedicine and telecare in Japan, *Journal of Telemedicine and Telecare*, **6**, 187–204, 2000

205. Lister G, *Global Health: Implications for Policy*, Nuffield Trust, London, 1999. See also the web page at http://www.nuffieldtrust.org.uk/health2/Lister.%20Policydoc.doc

206. Coyle D, *The Weightless World*, Capstone, Oxford, 1977, Chapter 10

207. Fujimoto M and Miyazaki K, Industrial innovation, government and society: telemedicine and telecare, *Science and Public Policy*, **27**, 347–366, 2000

208. Nitzkin J L, Zhu N and Marier R L, Reliability of telemedicine examination, *Telemedicine Journal*, **3**, 141–158, 1997

209. Coyle D, *The Weightless World*, Capstone, Oxford, 1977, Chapter 1

210. Sullivan-Trainor M, *Detour: The Truth About the Information Superhighway*, IDG, San Mateo, CA, 1994, Chapter 4

211. See the web site on Federal Telemedicine activities at http://www.cbloch.com

212. Randall N, *The Soul of the Internet*, Thomson, Boston, MA, Chapter 15

213. United States General Accounting Office, *Telemedicine—Federal Strategy Is Needed to Guide Investments*, Report NSIAD/HEHS-97-67. 02/14/97, Washington, DC, 1997. See the web page at http://www.gao.gov/openrecs97/abstracts/n397067.htm

214. Jones E, Sweeping GAO report urges cohesive telemedicine strategy, *Telemedicine and Telehealth Networks*, **3** (3), 11–12, 1997

215. Dakins D R, ASTP focuses on telemedicine business strategies, *Telemedicine and Telehealth Networks*, **3** (6), 19–21, 1997

216. American Telemedicine Association, *ATA Adopts Telehomecare Clinical Guidelines*. See the web page at http://www.atmeda.org/news/list.html

217. Interdisciplinary Telehealth Standards Working Group, *Report of the Interdisciplinary Telehealth Standards Working Group*. See the copy of the report at

the Arent Fox web page at http://www.arentfox.com/quickguide/businesslines/e-health/e-health_telemed/e-healthnewsalerts/telehlth/telehlth.html

218. Garfield M J T, *Knowledge Creation Using Telecommunications as a Tool: A Study of State Telemedicine Policy*, PhD Thesis, University of Georgia, 1999

219. Dakins D R, Hybrid business models rely on out-of-box thinking, *Telemedicine and Telehealth Networks*, **4** (2), 33–35, 1998

220. Crowe B L, *Telemedicine in Australia*, Australian Institute of Health and Welfare, Canberra, 1993

221. Mitchell J, *The Challenge to Embed Telepsychiatry*, John Mitchell and Associates, Adelaide, December 1994. See also http://www.jma.com.au/telepsyc.htm

222. Mitchell J, *Establishing Renal Clinical Medicine, Chapter 1: Description of Project and Management*, John Mitchell and Associates, Adelaide, September 1995. See also http://www.jma.com.au/tqehrep1.htm

223. Crowe B L, An overview of telemedicine development in Australia, *Informatics in Australia*, **6** (3), 85–88, 1997

224. House of Representatives Standing Committee on Family and Community Affairs, *Health On Line. A Report on Health Information Management and Telemedicine*, Parliament House, Canberra, 1997

225. Department of Health, *The Information Management and Technology (IM&T) Strategy for the NHS in England: Getting Better with Information*, HMSO, London, 1992

226. Curry R G, Norris A C and Parroy S, *Telemedical Activity in the United Kingdom: A Review and Assessment*, Department of Health Report: Contract DH121/6374, London, 1996

227. Curry R G, Norris A C, Parroy S and Melhuish P J, The strategic development and application of telemedicine, *Informatics in Australia*, **6** (3), 107–110, 1997

228. Curry R G and Norris A C, *A Review and Assessment of Telecare Activity in The UK and Recommendations for Development*, Department of Health Report: Contract DH 121/6523, London, 1997

229. NHS Executive, *Full LIS Guidance—Annex H: Telemedicine, Wetherby, 1999*. See also the web version at http://www.doh.gov.uk/nhsexipu/implemen/flis/guidance/annexes/annexh.htm

230. See the NHS Direct Internet page at http://www.doh.gov.uk/nhsexec/direct.htm

231. See the Cardiff University web site at http://www.cf.ac.uk/uwcc/masts/sirc/about.html

232. Multimedia Development Corporation, *Excerpts from the Speeches of Mahathir Mohamed on the Multimedia Super Corridor*, Pelanduk, Subang Jaya, 1998

233. Dakins D R, Malaysia report illuminates telemedicine standards, *Telemedicine and Telehealth Networks*, **3** (6), 7–8, 1997

234. Allen A and Wheeler T, The leaders: US programs doing more than 500 interactive consults in 1997, *Telemedicine Today*, **6** (3), 36–37, 1998

235. Taylor P, Evaluating telemedicine systems and services, in Wooton R and Craig J (eds) *Introduction to Telemedicine*, Royal Society of Medicine, London, 1999, Chapter 8

236. Vidmar D A, Plea for standardization in dermatology: a worm's eye view, *Telemedicine Journal*, **3**, 173–178, 1997

237. Gale M E, Vincent M E and Robbins A H, Teleradiology for remote diagnosis, a prospective multi-year evaluation, *Journal of Digital Imaging*, **10**, 47–50, 1997

238. Gerbert B, Maurer T, Berger T *et al*, Primary care physicians as gatekeepers in managed care: primary care physicians and dermatologists' skills at secondary prevention of skin cancer, *Archives of Dermatology*, **132**, 1030–1038, 1996

239. Harrison R, Clayton W and Wallace P, Can telemedicine be used to improve communication between primary and secondary care?, *British Medical Journal*, **313**, 333–335, 1996

240. Brecht R M, Gray C L, Peterson C and Youngblood B, The University of Texas Medical Branch—Texas Department of Criminal Justice: findings from the first year of operation, *Telemedicine Journal*, **2**, 7–9, 1996

241. American Institute of Medicine, *Telemedicine: A Guide to Assessing Telecommunications in Health Care*, See the summary report at the web site http://www.nap.edu/readingroom/books/telemed/summary.html

242. Mitchell J, *Mental Health Telemedicine Program*, John Mitchell and Associates, Adelaide, 1997

243. Elford R, White H, Bowering R, Ghandi A *et al*, A randomized, controlled trial of child psychiatric assessments conducted using videoconferencing, *Journal of Telemedicine and Telecare*, **6**, 73–82, 2000

244. Kvedar J C, Edwards R A, Menn E R *et al*, The substitution of digital images for dermatological physical consultation, *Archives of Dermatology*, **133**, 161–167, 1997

245. Stevens A, Milne R, Lilford, R and Gabbay J, Keeping pace with new technologies: systems needed to identify and evaluate them, *British Medical Journal*, **319**, 1291, 1999

246. Rosen R and Gabbay J, Linking health technology assessment to practice, *British Medical Journal*, **319**, 1292, 1999

247. Whitten P, Kingsley C and Grigsby J, Results of a meta-analysis of cost–benefit research: is this a question worth asking?, *Journal of Telemedicine and Telecare*, **6** (Suppl 1), 4–6, 2000

248. Mair F S, Haycox A, May C and Williams T, A review of telemedicine cost-effectiveness studies, *Journal of Telemedicine and Telecare*, **6** (Suppl 1), 38–40, 2000

249. Hakansson S and Gavelin C, What do we really know about the cost-effectiveness of telemedicine?, *Journal of Telemedicine and Telecare*, **6** (Suppl 1), 133–136, 2000

250. Togno J M, Lundin R, Buckley P and Hovel J, Rural health and IT&T in Australia—the results of qualitative and quantitative surveys of the needs, perceptions, and expectations of rural and remote health professionals, *Journal of Telemedicine and Telecare*, **2** (Suppl 1), 104–105, 1996

251. Mitchell J, *Establishing Renal Telemedicine: An Evaluation of the Queen Elizabeth Hospital Renal Dialysis Telemedicine Project 1994–1995, Chapter 8: Cost-Effectiveness*, John Mitchell and Associates, Adelaide, 1995. See also the excerpt of the report at the web site at http://www.jma.com.au/telemedupdate3.htm and other web-based chapters of the report referred to at this site

252. McIntosh E and Cairns J, A framework for the economic evaluation of telemedicine, *Journal of Telemedicine and Telecare*, **3** (3), 132–139, 1997

253. Hailey D, Jacobs P, Simpson J and Doze S, An assessment framework for telemedicine applications, *Journal of Telemedicine and Telecare*, **5** (3), 162–170, 1999

254. Mitchell J, Increasing the cost-effectiveness of telemedicine by embracing e-health, *Journal of Telemedicine and Telecare*, **6** (Suppl 1), 16–19, 2000

255. The following web page describes a CD-ROM that you can buy to help you 'build your own telemedicine program successfully': http://www.galvaniinteractive.com/portfolio/UVM_TM_980322/introduction/body_frame.html

256. Doolittle G C and Cook D, Defining the needs of a telemedicine service, in

Wootton R and Craig J (eds) *Introduction to Telemedicine*, Royal Society of Medicine, London, 1999, Chapter 6

257. Jabelian S T, *Impact of Telemedicine on Rural Communities: Tatamagouche, a Case Study (Nova Scotia)*, MURP Thesis, Daltech-Dalhousie University, 1997

258. Tachakra S, The changes patients expect to result from telemedicine, *Journal of Telemedicine and Telecare*, **6**, 295–300, 2000

259. Chuang D, *Client Acceptance of Telemedicine*, PhD Thesis, University of Michigan, 1997

260. Clyburn C A, *An Integrated Process Re-engineering Model for Improving Health Care Delivery Using Telemedicine*. This very interesting article was available at the web site http://www.matmo.org/pages/library/papers/reengineer/procreng.html but the link is now inactive and all attempts to recover it have failed. See http://www.tatrc.org/ for contact details.

261. Bentley C, *Introducing PRINCE*, NCC Blackwell, Oxford, 1992

262. Hammer M and Champy J, *Re-engineering the Corporation*, Brearley, London, 1993

263. Bharadwaj V, *Web Based Workflow in Secure Collaborative Telemedicine*, MS Thesis, West Virginia University, 2000

264. Tachakra S, Colour perception in telemedicine, *Journal of Telemedicine and Telecare*, **5**, 211–219, 1999

265. Dawson J A, Cohen D, Candelier C *et al*, Domiciliary midwifery support in high-risk pregnancy incorporating telephonic fetal heart rate monitoring: a health technology randomized assessment, *Journal of Telemedicine and Telecare*, **5**, 220–230, 1999

266. Hu P J-H, *Management of Telemedicine Technology in Healthcare Organizations: Technology Acceptance, Adoption, Evaluation, and their Implications*, PhD Thesis, University of Arizona, 1998

267. American Medical Association, *CME Resource Guide: Chapter 7, Section 2: The Promotion of Quality Telemedicine, Part II*, 1996. See the web version of the report at http://www.ama-assn.org/cmeselec/cmeres/cme-7-2.htm

268. See, for example, the summary of the Malaysian Telemedicine Bill (1997) at the Arent Fox web site at http://www.arentfox.com/quickguide/businesslines/e-health/e-health_telemed/e-healthnewsalerts/malaysian_telemed_bill/malaysian_telemed_bill.html

269. Tomenson J A and Paddle G M, Better quality studies through review of protocols, *Journal of Occupational Medicine*, **33**, 1240–1243, 1991

270. Berg M, Working with protocols: a sociological view, *Netherlands Journal of Medicine*, **3**, 119–125, 1996

271. Stanberry B A, *The Legal and Ethical Aspects of Telemedicine*, Royal Society of Medicine, London, 1998, Chapter 5

272. Fombrun S, *Turning Points: Creating Change in Corporations*, McGraw-Hill, New York, 1992

273. Kanter R M, *The Change Masters: Corporate Entrepreneurs at Work*, Allen & Unwin, London, 1984

274. Warisse J M, *Communicative Implications of Implementing Telemedicine Technology: A Framework of Telecompetence*, PhD Thesis, Ohio State University, 1996

275. Leitner P J, Innovations create ripe climate for mainstream telemedicine adoption, *Telemedicine and Telehealth Networks*, **4** (1), 31–34, 1998

276. British Medical Association, *Medical Ethics Today: Its Practice and Philosophy*, BMJ Publishing Group, London, 1993

277. NHSE, *Report on the Review of Patient-Identifiable Information*, The Caldicott

Report, Department of Health, 1997. See also the web-based version of the report at http://www.doh.gov.uk/confiden/back.htm

278. Kelly K, Patient data, confidentiality, and electronics, *British Medical Journal*, **316**, 718–719, 1998

279. New Zealand Health Information Service, *Health Information Privacy and Confidentiality*, New Zealand Health Information Service, Wellington, 1995. See the web version at http://www.nzhis.govt.nz/publications/Privacy.html

280. Klein S R and Manning W L, Telemedicine and the law, *Journal of the Healthcare Information and Management Systems Society*, **9** (3), 35–40, 1995. See the updated web version at http://www.netreach.net/~wmanning/telmedar.htm

281. Dyer C, BMA's patient confidentiality rules are deemed unlawful, *British Medical Journal*, **319**, 1221, 1999. See the web version at http://www.bmj.com/cgi/content/full/319/7219/1221/a

282. Hodge J G, Goslin L O and Jacobson P D, Legal issues concerning electronic health information: privacy, quality and liability, *Journal of the American Medical Association (Health Law and Ethics)*, **282** (15), 1466–1471, 1999. See the web version at http://jama.ama-assn.org/issues/v282n15/rfull/jlm80037.html

283. Cheong I R, Privacy and security of personal health information, *Journal of Informatics in Primary Care*, 15–17 March, 1996. See the web version at http://www.schin.ncl.ac.uk/phcsg/informatics/mar96/mar5.htm

284. General Medical Council, *Duties of a Doctor—Confidentiality: Guidance from the General Medical Council*, General Medical Council, London, 1995

285. The Health Law Resource, *S.1360—Medical Records Confidentiality Act of 1995*. See the summary at the web site http://www.netreach.net/~wmanning/s1360dig.htm

286. National Library of Medicine, *CBM95-10: Confidentiality of Electronic Health Data: 1990–1996*, Bethesda, MD, 1996

287. Stanberry B A, *The Legal and Ethical Aspects of Telemedicine*, Royal Society of Medicine, London, 1998, Chapter 3

288. Lee-Winser J, The Data Protection Act: a decade of data protection in the NHS, *British Journal of Healthcare Computing and Information Management*, **12** (5), 20–21, 1995

289. Barber B, Skerman P and Saldanha R, Towards a measure of privacy, *British Journal of Healthcare Computing and Information Management*, **13** (5), 41, 1996

290. Yeates D and Cadle J, *Project Management for Information Systems*, 2nd edn, Pitman, London, 1996, Chapter 13

291. Greer T, *Understanding Intranets*, Microsoft Press, Redmond, 1998, Chapter 4

292. Molteno B, Is our clinical information safe?, *British Journal of Healthcare Computing and Information Management*, **13** (2), 40, 1996 (and editorial columns on page 6 of the same issue)

293. NHS Executive, *A Strategy for NHS-wide Networking*, Department of Health, London, 1994

294. NHS Executive, *NHS-wide Networking Programme Security Project*, Department of Health, London, 1995

295. Roscoe T J and Wells M, NHSnet—learning from academia, *British Medical Journal*, **318**, 377–379, 1999

296. De Lusignan S and Brown A, Internet can be accessed from NHSnet, *British Medical Journal*, **317**, 1319, 1998

297. Krol E and Ferguson P, *The Whole Internet for Windows 95*, O'Reilly, Sebastopol, CA, 1995, Chapter 14. You can get a copy of PGP from the web site http://web.mit.edu/network/pgp.html

298. American Bar Association Section of Science and Technology Information

Security Committee, *Digital Signature Guidelines Tutorial*. See the article at http://www.abanet.org/scitech/ec/isc/dsg-tutorial.html

299. Howard G S, *Introduction to Internet Security*, Prima Publishing, Roseville, CA, 1995

300. Taylor H, *Explosive Growth of Hypochondria Continues*, Harris Poll 44, 11 August, 2000, Harris Interactive, Rochester, NY, 2000. See web summary at http://www.harrisinteractive.com/harris_poll/index.asp?PID=104

301. Kassirer J P, Patients, physicians and the Internet, *Health Affairs*, **19** (6), 115–123, 2000. See the web version at http://www.medscape.com/ProjHope/HA/2000/v19.n06/ha1906.02.kass/ha1906.02.kass-01.html

302. Ludwig B and McMullin K, *Significant Technological Barriers for Healthcare on the Internet*. See National Academies web site at http://www4.nationalacademies.org/news.nsf/isbn/0309068436?OpenDocument

303. Binns K, Zapart K, Blyth B *et al*, *Ethics and the Internet*, Study 12950, Harris Interactive, Rochester, NY, 2000. Access the PDF version at the Internet Health Coalition web site at http://www.ihealthcoalition.org/content/Harris_report2000.pdf

304. King S A and Poulos S T, Ethical guidelines for on-line therapy in Fink J (ed), *How to Use Computers and Cyberspace in Clinical Practice of Psychotherapy*, Aronson, Leonia, NJ, 1999, pp 121–132

305. Meinhardt R A, New 'E-sign' law enables electronic prescriptions, *Drug Benefit Trends*, **12** (9), 23–24, 2000. See the web version at http://managedcare.medscape.com/SCP/DBT/2000/v12.n09/d1209.04.mein/d1209.04.mein-01.html

306. Winker M A, Flanagin A, Chi-Lum B *et al*, Guidelines for medical and health information sites on the Internet, *Journal of the American Medical Association*, **283** (12), 1600–1606, 2000

307. Health Internet Ethics web site, *Ethical Principles for Offering Internet Health Services to Customers*. See web site at http://www.hiethics.org/Principles/index.asp

308. Stanberry B A, *The Legal and Ethical Aspects of Telemedicine*, Royal Society of Medicine, London, 1998, Chapter 5

309. Powers M J and Harris N H, *Medical Negligence*, 2nd edn, Butterworths, London, 1994, pp 587–588

310. Stanberry B A, *The Legal and Ethical Aspects of Telemedicine*, Royal Society of Medicine, London, 1998, Chapter 6

311. Salter B, *The Politics of Change in the Health Service*, Macmillan, Basingstoke, 1998, Chapter 5

312. General Medical Council, *Professional Conduct and Practice: Fitness to Practise*, General Medical Council, London 1993

313. Stanberry B A, *The Legal and Ethical Aspects of Telemedicine*, Royal Society of Medicine, London, 1998, Chapter 7

314. Craig J O M C, Litigation concerning clinical radiology, in Powers M J and Harris N H (eds) *Medical Negligence*, 2nd edn, Butterworths, London, 1994, Chapter 41

315. Vincent C F, Driscoll P A *et al*, Accuracy of detection of radiography anomalies, *Archives of Emergency Medicine*, **5**, 101–109, 1988

316. Picot J, Meeting the need for educational standards in the practice of telemedicine and telehealth, *Journal of Telemedicine and Telecare*, **6** (Suppl 2), 59–62, 2000

317. Stanberry B A, *The Legal and Ethical Aspects of Telemedicine*, Royal Society of Medicine, London, 1998, Chapter 9

318. Shotwell L F, Technology adoption poses catch-22 for providers, *Telemedicine*

and Telehealth Networks, **2** (2), 1996. See the web page at http://arentfox.com/quickGuide/businessLines/e-health/e-health_telemed/e-healthNewsAlerts/tamingliab/tamingliab.html

319. Stanberry B, Rossignol G and Menke P, Contracting with health-care customers and specialists for the provision of telemedicine services across European borders: the TEN-Telemed legal project, *Journal of Telemedicine and Telecare*, **6** (Suppl 1), 104–106, 2000

320. Rogers R and Reardon J (eds), *Barriers to a Global Information Society for Health: Recommendations for International Action*, Report from the project G8-ENABLE, European Commission Information Society Project Office, Brussels, December 1998. See also the web pages at: http://www.ehto.be/sp5

321. Waters R J, *Health Information Systems and Telemedicine*, Arent Fox, Washington, DC, 1995. See the web version at http://arentfox.com/quickguide/businesslines/e-health/e-health_telemed/e-healthnewsalerts/licenseimplic/licenseimplic.html

322. Nohr L E, Global medicine and licensing, *Journal of Telemedicine and Telecare*, **6** (Suppl 1), 170–172, 2000

323. American Medical Association, *CME Resource Guide: Chapter 7, Section 4: The Physician Licensure Debate on Telemedicine: An Update*, US Medical Licensure Statistics and Current Licensure Requirements, 1997. See the web version of the report at http://www.ama-assn.org/cmeselec/cmeres/cme-7-4.htm

324. Gobis L, An overview of state laws and approaches to mimimize licensure barriers, *Telemedicine Today*, **5** (6), 14, 15, 18, 1997.

325. See, for example, the text of the Maastricht Treaty at http://europa.eu.int/en/record/mt/top.html

326. Lapolla M and Millis B, Is telemedicine reimbursement a real barrier or a convenient straw man?, *Telemedicine Today*, **5** (6), 5, 1997

327. Hart T and Fazzini L, *Intellectual Property Law*, Macmillan, Basingstoke, 1997

328. Stanberry B A, *The Legal and Ethical Aspects of Telemedicine*, Royal Society of Medicine, London, 1998, Chapter 8

329. Albert J, *The Copyrightability of Factual Compilations Such as Databases Containing Medical Records*, Arent Fox, Washington, DC, 2000. See the article at the web site http://www.arentfox.com/quickGuide/businessLines/e-health/e-health_telemed/e-healthNewsAlerts/cpyrtmeddata/cpyrtmeddata.html

INDEX